Text Copyright © 2018 Gregory L. Smith

All Right Reserved

The Anti-Munchies Appetite Killer

tetrahydrocannabivarin (THCV)

THCV, the abbreviation for tetrahydrocannabivarin, is an extract from hemp oil. Much like CBD, it does not cause euphoria, or get people "high". It is also legal and available in all 50 states without a prescription, and it has many health benefits that are entirely different from CBD. I call it CBD*plus* is this book, so that it does not get confused with THC, or tetrahydrocannabinol, which is the component of medical cannabis that causes euphoria as well as addiction and requires physician supervision.

CBD*plus* has a proven impact on:

Weight loss

Pre-diabetes

Diabetes

High blood lipids

Fatty liver disease

Metabolic syndrome

Learn more ...

Get Off Opioids! ©

Coming Soon!

By Gregory L. Smith, MD, MPH

Cannabidiol (CBD): What You Need to Know ©

Available on Amazon!

By Gregory L. Smith, MD, MPH

To learn more or for specific questions regarding tetrahydrocannabivarin (CBD*plus*), cannabidiol (CBD) and medical cannabis, contact Dr. Gregory Smith directly at MedicalMarijuana@Mail.com

Or visit his website:

http://www.cannabis-md.com

Dedication:

To all of those who have taken the time, energy, and oftentimes leaps of faith, to bring *cannabis sativa* out of its state of scientific suspended animation and back into our medicine cabinets.

Thank you.

Disclaimer:

The information provided in this book is current and vetted as of June 2018. The research and new data coming out about *cannabis sativa* and tetrahydrocannabivarin (CBD*plus* or THCV) and cannabidivarin (CBDV) is certain to change. This book is intended to give the reader a baseline framework, to which they can add additional information as it comes along in the future.

TABLE OF CONTENTS:

Preface 6

Chapter 1: What is CBD*plus*? (THCV) 21

Chapter 2: History and Legal Issues of Hemp Oil Use 36

Chapter 3: How Does CBD*plus* Work? 50

Chapter 4: How Safe is CBD*plus*? 83

Chapter 5: How to Use CBD*plus* 95

Chapter 6: Diabetes MELLITUS 107

Chapter 7: High Cholesterol and BLOOD Lipids ... 116

Chapter 8: Weight Loss 122

Chapter 9: Fatty Liver Disease 148

Chapter 10: Metabolic Syndrome 155

Chapter 11: Preventive Doses of CBD*plus* 161

Abbreviations 165

Index 168

PREFACE

The Medical Cannabis Refugee

I want to share one powerful story that was a major motivator for me to write this book. My textbook for medical professionals came out about a year ago, and I was invited to a large medical cannabis convention in Boston to give a lecture on how to use cannabidiol (CBD) and tetrahydrocannabivarin (CBD*plus*) as treatments for a variety of conditions.

After the lecture, I was invited to do a book signing for two hours. I love book signings because they give me an opportunity to get close and personal with those who have read my book. During this particular occasion, a young mother approached me to buy my book. She explained to me the hardships of moving from North Carolina to Colorado, so that she could obtain medical cannabis for her daughter, who suffers from intractable seizures.

She expressed that she was able to get CBD oil in North Carolina by having it shipped legally to her home; however, her daughter's specific case of epilepsy had a minimal response to the CBD only oil.

Thankfully, she was able to obtain a small quantity of whole-plant medical cannabis that contains high levels of the ingredient THCV, or CBD*plus*. Upon introducing this ingredient to the treatment, this young mother quickly learned that her daughter's seizures have almost disappeared—noting a significant reduction from dozens every week, to nearly singular episodes every month or so.

She also found that rubbing pure tetrahydrocannabinol (THC) oil inside her daughter's mouth right after a seizure helped her recover much faster from their severe aftereffects.

Since whole-plant cannabis is considered a criminal offense in North Carolina, this young mother decided that is was time to weigh her options; and after discussing the benefits with her husband, the young couple thought it would be best for their daughter to move the family to Colorado—where convenient and legal access to CBD, THC, and CBD*plus* is a way of life.

I believe that this family's experience is an important anecdote to consider for many reasons. Not only does their story highlight how CBD can be an excellent medication by itself for several conditions, it also draws attention to the fact that it is sometimes it not enough and depends on the individual.

Therefore, it is essential for both doctors and patients to have access to all of the wonderful oils and ingredients in cannabis—not just CBD alone. And ultimately, sharing this tale with others gives me a chance to educate patients and family members, in a relatable context, on the numerous beneficial resources that are out there—as well as to provide support, ideas, feedback and advice.

Within each chapter, I have provided a number of educational websites that I, myself, have found to be particularly useful to patients, family members and caregivers.

Alphabet Soups of Initials

Before we delve too far into the meat of the book, it's a good idea to go ahead and get the long list of funny names and similar sounding initials figured out. All of these names and initials refer to oils that are in the plant *cannabis sativa*. There are over 300 distinct oils in hemp oil, and about 100 of them are medically active cannabinoids.

Being a cannabinoid means that the oil works with the Endocannabinoid System (ECS) that is in our brain and bodies. The two most common cannabinoids are tetrahydrocannabinol (THC) and cannabidiol (CBD). THC is essentially the only oil that causes an individual to get high.

All of the other 99+ cannabinoids can have various therapeutic effects on a myriad of medical conditions, but they do not cause euphoria or the sensation of "getting high."

CBD is the oil that is taking the country by storm right now due to the many beneficial effects is has on pain, degenerative conditions—such as arthritis—and even helps with weaning off opioids.

CBD is a very safe oil, which I explain to doctors when giving lecture on how to use hemp oil. CBD is actually so safe that it can be sold next to the olive oil in grocery stores. If you'd like to learn more about the many benefits of CBD, I recommend my book, *CBD: What You Need to Know* (Kindle Publishing 2017), available on Amazon.

CBD*plus*

This book is about neither THC or CBD; it is about another amazing oil from the *cannabis sativa* plant, which I have come to call "CBD*plus*". The real scientific name for CBD*plus* is tetrahydrocannabivarin, which, phonetically pronounced, is Tetra-Hydro-Canna-Biv-arin.

As you can see, this long and hard to pronounce oil does not have a very easy or convenient name. The official abbreviation for tetrahydrocannabivarin is THCV; neither of which are very useful, considering the likeness to THC, or tetrahydrocannabinol.

THC is the oil in cannabis that causes euphoria, which is also known as "getting high", and is often associated with many unpleasant side-effects and drug dependency.

THCV—or as I call it in this book, CBD*plus*—does not cause euphoria, and is not associated with significant side-effects or drug dependency. In many ways, CBD*plus* is considered to be much like CBD; however, it has a number of potent medical benefits that make it entirely different from CBD.

CBD and THC

THC and CBD are the two oils in *cannabis sativa* that are in the highest concentration. Medical cannabis plants can have as much as 25% THC or CBD in them by dry weight.

They are literally dripping with the oil. However, hemp oil is derived from cannabis plants that are very low in THC, less than 0.3%. This is because there is essentially no THC in hemp oil that it is legal, over-the-counter and very safe to use. Being less than

0.3% THC means that you cannot get high from using hemp oil, or from products derived from it.

Hemp oil products still need to be tested in order to ensure that they don't contain THC. The other 99+ cannabinoids are known as 'minor cannabinoids', because only very tiny amounts of any one of these oils are found in hemp oil, usually.

Most of these minor cannabinoids represent less than ½ percent of the oil, and it's only been in the past few years that enough of these oils have been extracted to be able to conduct further research. From this recent research, however, there have been some amazing findings.

Tetrahydrocannabivarin (THCV or CBD*plus*) is one of the minor cannabinoids. Most scientific texts use the abbreviation THCV, but this can get easily confused with THC and all of the bad press associated with THC. Truth be told, CBD*plus* is actually the exact opposite of THC.

There is absolutely no associated euphoria, and it reduces hunger as well. Studies have shown that long term use of appropriate doses of CBD*plus* can result in several positive effects on one's health.

Another minor cannabinoid oil with similar properties to CBD*plus* is cannabidivarin (Canna-Bid-ivarin), abbreviated as CBDV.

CBDV is currently being evaluated by a large pharmaceutical company because of its many wonderful health effects; and within the next couple of years, we will be hearing about the amazing antibiotic properties of cannabichromene (Canna-Bi-Chro-mean), abbreviated as CBC, and cannabigerol (Canna-Bij-erol), abbreviated as CBG.

When THC is allowed to age, it will turn into another oil called cannabinol (Canna-Bin-ol), abbreviated as CBN, and has its own complete set of medical properties.

When the plant is freshly cut all, of the many oils in the plant are in their acidic form—which is expressed with a small letter 'a' after then name (for example, CBDa and THCa)—and with time or heating, the acidic forms convert to the decarboxylated forms that we commonly known as THC, CBD, and CBD*plus*. Oftentimes, the acidic forms of these oils act very differently in the body compared to the decarboxylated forms. For example, THCa in fresh cannabis oil does not cause euphoria.

Cannabis or Marijuana?

Personally, I try to keep away from the politics that surround the topic of *cannabis sativa*; however, there is an important history lesson to be learned about the use of the word 'cannabis.' Prior to the prohibition of alcohol in 1919 in the US, the only form of *cannabis sativa* that most of the population knew about was cannabis extract.

In fact, during that time there were thousands of products containing cannabis extract that were readily available as an over-the-counter remedy and were used to treat a myriad of medical conditions.

Owing to the prohibition of alcohol in 1919, people began searching for alternative ways to produce the euphoric intoxication often associated with alcohol. It wasn't long before the middle-class of the U.S. discovered the euphoric aftereffects of smoking cannabis bud. Prior to this time period, smoking cannabis was only common among Mexican migrant workers and within the jazz music scene.

It wasn't until the 19030's, with the crossover of jazz music into mainstream America, that smoking cannabis became a rather common occurrence—primarily because alcohol was illegal by federal law at the time—and ultimately led to the cultural merging of black jazz musicians with the jazz aficionados of 'white' America.

Although this may be, the integration of the 'races' would eventually spur significant social and political backlash; beginning with a series of propagandist anti-cannabis films—namely "Refer Madness"—in which white women were often portrayed as having transformed into sexual beasts upon consorting with black men.

In the wake of this complex social phenomenon, the U.S. government would soon pass The Marihuana Tax Act of 1937; which largely outlawed the recreational use of cannabis throughout the country. Interestingly enough, the federal legislators responsible for drafting the act were already aware of the increasing popularity of *cannabis sativa* among the general public, having considered that cannabis extracts were the second most common prescribed ingredient in pharmaceuticals at the time.

Regardless of general preference during the time, federal legislators sought to vilify cannabis by fostering a negative public image in association with the Spanish term *Marihuana* (spelling is later changed to *marijuana*, with a 'j')—an expression that translates to "Mary Jane"—which was first used by Mexican migrant workers when referring to cannabis.

In order to adversely influence the country's stance on cannabis, the legislators wanted to bring attention to an unfavorable correlation between recreational smoking and poor Mexican migrant workers, which would thereby denigrate cannabis around the U.S.

For this reason and in my own attempt to rid racist terminology from our culture and language, I will be using the correct term 'cannabis' throughout this book.

So, You Want to Learn About CBD*plus*

Perhaps you've heard about the exciting and novel medical benefits of medical cannabis, but you're concerned about "getting high" or "addicted" to the THC that is found in whole-plant cannabis.

Or perhaps you live in a state or country where whole-plant cannabis hasn't been legalized, even though CBD*plus* can be obtained easily and legally, and now you're interested in finding out if it could be beneficial to you.

Perhaps you have a family member or loved one that has a medical condition—such as high blood fats, diabetes, or obesity—that could potentially respond to CBD*plus*; and now, you want to learn more about how CBD*plus* works and how to use it.

Or perhaps you have already had an opportunity to see how CBD*plus* can work and want to get a deeper understanding of it altogether.

Finally, you may have noticed that CBD*plus* oils and extracts are available without a prescription at stores and online and want to know why sometimes a doctor's visit isn't required to get CBD*plus*.

Unfortunately, you can't ask over 95% of doctors or pharmacists about CBD*plus*, because they have had no formal training on medical cannabis, CBD*plus*, CBD or even the Endocannabinoid System within the body.

Written by the Author of the #1 Selling Medical Cannabis Textbook

My name is Dr. Gregory L. Smith, and I am a Harvard-trained physician with extensive residency experience who is board certified in Preventive Medicine. I have been in primary care practice for over 30 years. About 15 years ago, I took a course on how to use cannabis medically for a variety of conditions. It occurred to me that there was no science-based textbook about medical cannabis from which medical students and physicians can learn. If a medical professional wanted to learn about medical cannabis, they had to painstakingly research each subject or condition, read studies, and clinical anecdotes—many of them decades old.

To address the lack of data at the time, I would go on to spend two and a half years gathering all of the available research on medical cannabis—including basic science research in animals, as well as tissue cultures and clinical trials in humans. I synthesized this body of information and wrote a medical textbook called, *Medical Cannabis: Basic Science and Clinical Applications*, which came out in early 2016 and is now a best seller among physicians, medical students, nurses, pharmacists and caregivers.

> For more information or to buy the textbook:
> https://www.aylesburypress.com/

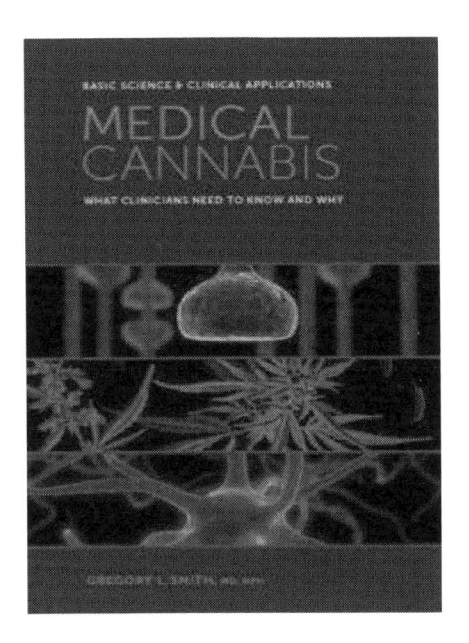

Strong Resistance from Physicians

Within a few months of publishing my textbook, I realized that most physicians and medical organizations like the American Medical Association, were still very much against medical cannabis. They felt that there was not enough research to recommend it as a serious medication. There was also still a strong feeling among my fellow physicians that medical cannabis laws were just a means to bypass the prohibition against using cannabis for recreational purposes. This stubborn resistance to medical cannabis is changing—but very slowly.

In the Spring of 2017, the National Academies of Sciences released a very important article, *The Health Effects of Cannabis and Cannabinoids: The*

Current State of Evidence and Recommendations for Research'. This large group of health care providers, and scientists reviewed 10,000's of cases of scientific research and found that medical cannabis was effective for several conditions and that it may be effective in many more; however, research has been significantly hindered by the federal government for the past 40 years.

Profit Motivation from Pharmaceutical Companies

There is very little profit motivation among the larger pharmaceutical companies to spend the millions of dollars it requires to get high quality, cannabis-based pharmaceuticals approved by the FDA. The main active ingredients of all cannabis-based medications will be THC, CBD, and/or CBD*plus*. Cannabinoids are naturally occurring plant-based compounds, for which patents have been prohibited within the industry of big pharma.

Though this may be, a pharmaceutical company could easily imitate, rebrand and patent a cannabis-based medication already patented by a competitor—all without having to worry about patent infringement. Without patents such as these, several companies and businesses in the pharmaceutical industry would have a difficult time profiting from medications such as these.

Smaller, more focused pharmaceutical companies, such as G.W. Pharmaceuticals from the U.K., have approved a number of pharmaceuticals in several countries and have been pending FDA approval in the U.S. for two separate drugs. It's quite interesting to note that the first FDA approval concerning medical cannabis might soon be for a pharmaceutical called

Epidiolex®; a brand-named drug designed to help those suffering from intractable childhood seizures; costing anywhere from $1200-$1800 each month.

This new drug is 99% CBD oil extracted from a specific strain of medical cannabis only. You can also find similar 99% CBD extracts and products both online and in stores for around $100-$200 each month—no prescription necessary. On the downside, however; considering the unlikelihood of Epidiolex® receiving FDA approval, it's probably safe to assume that, without it, the drug won't be covered through health insurance either.

How to Educate Your Physician

Physicians are accustomed to being in control of the patient-physician relationship and having all of the answers—which can create a significant problem. Nearly 95% of physicians have never taken a class on the Endocannabinoid System (ECS) or have ever learned anything in medical school or residency about using THC and CBD*plus*. I have been told by several medical school deans that they are worried about losing federal funding to the medical school if they teach anything about *cannabis sativa*, including hemp oil derived medications.

Although this is changing over time, it will probably be several years before a sizable percentage of physicians and pharmacists have a good working knowledge of medical cannabis or CBD*plus*.

The following is website that provides a nice quick summary of the 'pros' and 'cons' of medical cannabis. I have found that if I can get a physician to read this summary, I can quickly get them motivated and excited to learn more.

> Ask your doctor and read this quick and concise article called
>
> "The 10-Minute Summary," at ProCon.org.
>
> (http://medicalcannabis.procon.org/view.resource.php?resourceID=142)

Empowering People

While the use of CBD*plus* is slowly filtering into the medical community, small profit motivated pharmaceutical companies are moving ahead with high cost medical cannabis preparations, and I felt a strong need to write a concise book that will empower people to take hold of their right to have access to CBD*plus*—a legal, effective and very safe medication. After decades of minimal research, there are now many studies on CBD*plus*, CBD, and THC and cannabinoids ongoing at this time.

CBD*plus* is Available Without a Prescription in All 50 States:

It is also important to learn how and why CBD and CBD*plus* are legal and available without a prescription in all 50 states. Even though most people think they have to visit a physician and be in a state-run cannabis registry to get CBD*plus*, this is not true.

This book will tell you how to make sure that you are getting high quality and safe CBD*plus* products. Laws can change, and the current regressive approach on CBD*plus* coming out of Washington may lead to limitations on our access to it.

Therefore, when you decide to purchase CBD*plus*, do some research beforehand in order to make sure that it is legal in your state or country.

Section I:

What you need to know about CBD*plus*

CHAPTER 1: WHAT IS CBD*PLUS*? (THCV)

CBD*plus* is an oil found in the *cannabis sativa* plant and is comparable to CBD; neither produce any euphoric effects—meaning, it will not get you 'high'— unlike THC, the most well-known ingredient of cannabis. CBD*plus* is only found in tiny amounts in most strain of cannabis flowers or buds. It is also present to a much lesser degree in the stems and stalks of the plant.

CBD*plus* is found in higher concentrations in only a few hard to get strains of the plant, and barely present in most strains. It is one of over 100 cannabinoid oils that can be found only in the cannabis plant. CBD, cannabigerol (CBG) and THC are the three cannabinoids found in large quantities in cannabis, while many others found in only minute quantities in the plant.

Dozens of other oils besides CBD, CBG, and THC are only found in tiny amounts in the cannabis plant and are referred to as 'minor cannabinoids'.

21

Owing to the legal constraints against studying extracts from cannabis, there is very little research or information about the minor cannabinoids.

Later in the chapter, I have provided a list of many of the other lesser cannabinoids with their potential health benefits. Over the next few years we can expect more research on the health benefits of these other cannabinoids.

Although this book is about CBD*plus* (THCV), I will first give a brief introduction to hemp oil and medical cannabis in general.

Hemp vs. Cannabis:

> There is surprisingly a considerable amount of confusion among people intimately involved with cannabis—especially concerning the difference between hemp and cannabis. The difference between the two is very important. When CBD*plus* oil made in the U.S. is extracted from research-based hemp plants (less than 0.3% THC), it is considered a nutritional supplement that is legal and available over-the-counter in all 50 states.
>
> However, when the same CBD*plus* oil is extracted from non-research-based *cannabis sativa* plants, it is considered a Schedule I drug with significant criminal consequences. Thus, the exact same oil can be either an over-the-counter nutritional supplement or a Class I narcotic, along with heroin, LSD, and PCP. There is no medical or scientific reason for this—only politics and financial incentives of powerful pharmaceutical companies.

> Both hemp and cannabis are derived from the *cannabis sativa* plant. It was arbitrarily decided that if *cannabis sativa* that is less than 0.3% THC by weight, it is hemp and if it is over 0.3% THC then it is cannabis. Hemp has historically been used for millennia for industrial purposes. The plant fiber is used for fabric and rope, and the hemp oil for nutritional and industrial purposes. Whereas, cannabis is used for the oils from the flower or bud, for medical or recreational purposes.
>
> In summary, hemp oil is that which is extracted from the non-euphoric *cannabis sativa* plant, which is high in CBD, CBD*plus*, and very low in THC. CBD*plus* oil is a hemp oil that has been further extracted and refined so that there are even higher levels of CBD*plus* (3%-99%) and less of the other cannabinoid and terpene oils.

Subtypes of Cannabis Sativa

There are two medically important subtypes of *cannabis sativa*, which include *c. sativa sativa* and *c. sativa indica*. Sativa plants are tall and thin with long thin leaves; whereas, indica plants are short and stout with short wide leaves.

The image on page 25, from www.Leafscience.com, shows the physical differences of the two subtypes. The ruderalis subtype is not medically important. Historically, sativa and indica flourished in more southern parts of the world.

The sativa strains typically have high levels of CBD and very low levels of THC, whereas indica strains have the opposite, with much more potent levels of THC than CBD.

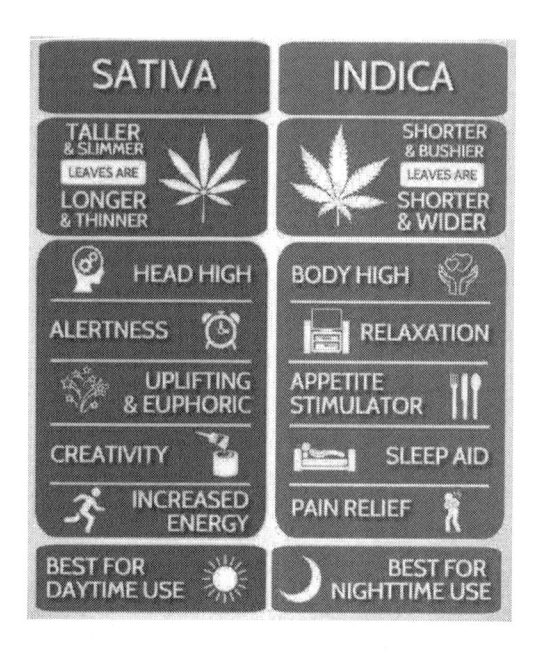

SATIVA	INDICA
TALLER & SLIMMER	SHORTER & BUSHIER
LEAVES ARE LONGER & THINNER	LEAVES ARE SHORTER & WIDER
HEAD HIGH	BODY HIGH
ALERTNESS	RELAXATION
UPLIFTING & EUPHORIC	APPETITE STIMULATOR
CREATIVITY	SLEEP AID
INCREASED ENERGY	PAIN RELIEF
BEST FOR DAYTIME USE	BEST FOR NIGHTTIME USE

In the past few decades, significant cross-breeding has led to the development of hundreds of different hybrid strains that have the characteristics of both subtypes.

Strains, colors and aromas do not provide any real information about how potent cannabis is—considering that THC, CBD, CBD*plus* all have zero odor. The only real way to know how much CBD*plus* or THC is in plant material is to have a laboratory test it.

Strains of Cannabis

There are literally hundreds of different strains of cannabis. There are strains that are based solely on the indica subtype, strains based on the sativa subtype, and the newer strains that are hybrids of both subtypes. These strains have comical and oftentimes entertaining names that are usually based on the fragrance or color of the crystals in the bud.

Some well know examples of strains include Maui Wowie, Blue Dream, Purple Haze and BC Bud. The variation in aromatic terpenes is a big factor in naming these strains, by adding color and odor to the 'bud.'

The amounts of THC, CBD, CBD*plus* and terpenes can vary significantly from batch to batch. Just because a strain was mild in the first batch, does not necessarily mean that the next batch that is grown will have the same potency. It is important to look at the laboratory test results from each batch prior to using each new batch of cannabis.

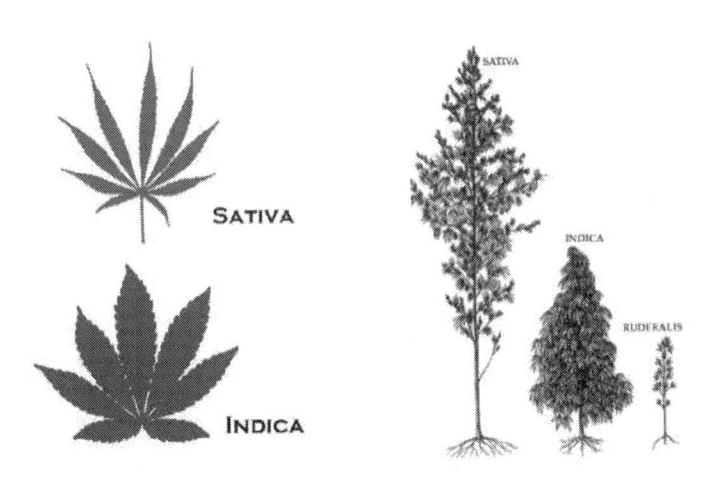

Medical vs. Recreational Cannabis

CBD has a much broader impact on health than THC. Some experts believe that 80% of the health benefits from cannabis come from CBD. Thus, cannabis that is to be used for medical purposes should usually be 1:1 ratio of CBD to THC or higher.

There are a few conditions where a higher ratio of THC to CBD is preferred. But generally, when the ratio of THC to CBD gets increased, so do the chances of getting 'high', addicted, or having side effects.

The Charlotte's web strain, developed in Colorado by the Stanley Brothers, has a ratio of 20:1 CBD*plus* and CBD, and less than 0.3% THC. This strain was specifically developed to treat intractable pediatric seizures. There are several other similar strains of high CBD that are very low THC cannabis.

Recreational strains of cannabis have much higher amounts of THC than CBD. Since CBD actually diminishes the euphoric effects of getting high, only very small amounts of CBD are usually found in these recreational strains. The most popular recreational strains of cannabis are often 18% or more THC and 0.2% CBD, giving a ratio of 1:90 CBD to THC.

Terpenes

In addition to the cannabinoids, there are several hundred terpenes that can be found in cannabis. Unlike cannabinoids, which are only found in cannabis, terpenes can be found in a wide variety of plants, herbs, fruits and vegetables.

It is often the terpenes that give different strains of cannabis their particular aroma and color. The terpenes are only present in a small amount in the plant oils, but many of the terpenes have their own health effects. However, only beta caryophyllene actually has health effects via one of the same receptors of the

Endocannabinoid System (ECS) that the cannabinoids use.

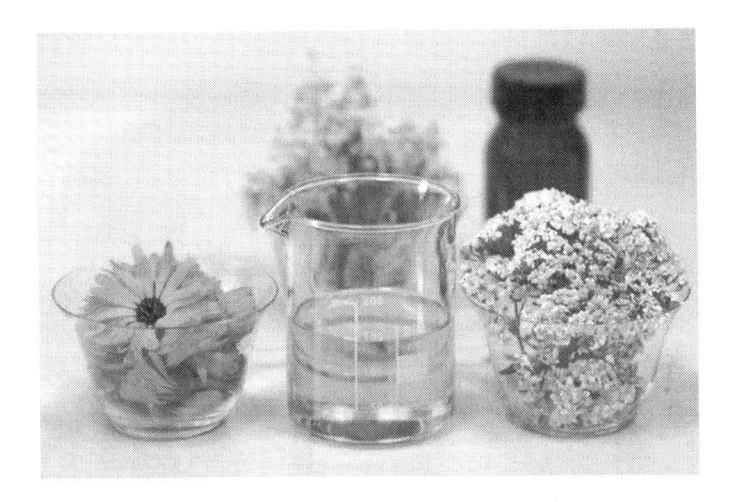

Beta caryophyllene is found in black pepper, hops, cloves and other plants. It does not cause the euphoria associated with THC, but is more similar to CBD and CBD*plus*, having several medically beneficial effects.

Only a handful of terpenes are known to be medically important, which I will discuss later on. All of the important terpenes are available over-the-counter individually as nutritional supplements.

There are over two hundred terpenes secreted in the same glands in the cannabis flower as the cannabinoids. These aromatic, often pungent oils found in plants, and herbs other than cannabis do not cause euphoria.

Although there has not been much research on terpenes to date, there is growing evidence to support medical benefits from several of the more common terpenes, which give different strains of cannabis characteristic fragrances and colors.

As was mentioned earlier, terpenes interact synergistically with cannabinoids as part of the Entourage Effect. Below I have provided information on some of the more common or important terpenes.

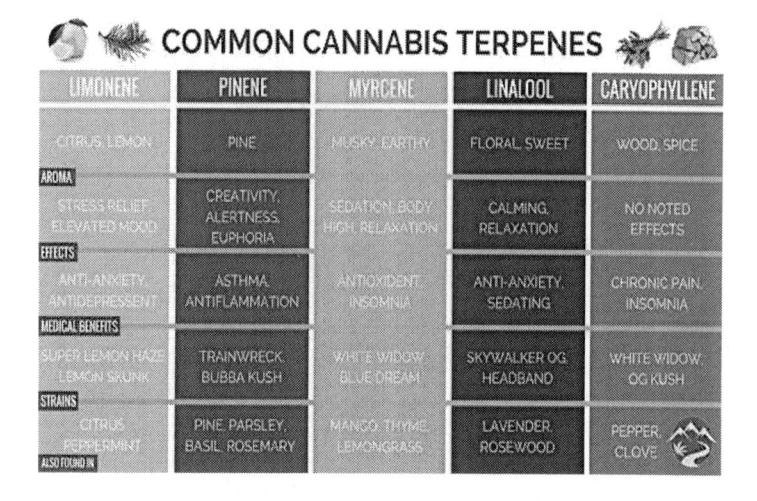

COMMON CANNABIS TERPENES

LIMONENE	PINENE	MYRCENE	LINALOOL	CARYOPHYLLENE
AROMA CITRUS, LEMON	PINE	MUSKY, EARTHY	FLORAL, SWEET	WOOD, SPICE
EFFECTS STRESS RELIEF, ELEVATED MOOD	CREATIVITY, ALERTNESS, EUPHORIA	SEDATION, BODY HIGH, RELAXATION	CALMING, RELAXATION	NO NOTED EFFECTS
MEDICAL BENEFITS ANTI-ANXIETY, ANTIDEPRESSENT	ASTHMA, ANTIFLAMMATION	ANTIOXIDENT, INSOMNIA	ANTI-ANXIETY, SEDATING	CHRONIC PAIN, INSOMNIA
STRAINS SUPER LEMON HAZE, LEMON SKUNK	TRAINWRECK, BUBBA KUSH	WHITE WIDOW, BLUE DREAM	SKYWALKER OG, HEADBAND	WHITE WIDOW, OG KUSH
ALSO FOUND IN CITRUS, PEPPERMINT	PINE, PARSLEY, BASIL, ROSEMARY	MANGO, THYME, LEMONGRASS	LAVENDER, ROSEWOOD	PEPPER, CLOVE

Caryophyllene:
    Smells like pepper or cloves. Also found in black pepper, cloves and cotton. Unlike any other terpene, it binds to CB2 cannabinoid receptors in the body.

Limonene:
    Smells like citrus. Also found in fruit rinds, peppermint and juniper. Has antifungal and antibacterial effects.

Myrcene:
    Smells like earthy cloves. Also found in mango, hops and lemongrass. Has sedating, muscle relaxing effects. Myrcene probably responsible for "in the couch" sensation.

Pinene:
    Smells like pine needles. Also found in pine, rosemary, basil, and parsley. Counteracts some adverse

effects of THC.

Flavonoids

Flavonoids are also present in cannabis oils, as well as all fruits and vegetables, and have potent anti-oxidant effects. In addition, they also contribute to the aroma and color of the plant.

The Entourage Effect

Whole-plant cannabis oil is made up of a combination of THC, CBD*plus*, other cannabinoids, as well as a wide array of terpenes and flavonoids.

In the 1980's, research conducted on pure synthetic THC analogues without any other cannabinoids or terpenes, has revealed that THC works better and in a much more natural way, with far fewer side effects, when other cannabinoids and terpenes are present.

The Entourage Effect
The synergy of various compounds in marijuana

- Cannabis contains several hundred compounds, including dozens of minor cannabinoids, various flavonoids, and terpenes (fragrant oils with medicinal properties).

- While many of these compounds have specific healing attributes, it is believed that when combined, the therapeutic impact of the whole plant is greater than the sum of its single-molecule parts.

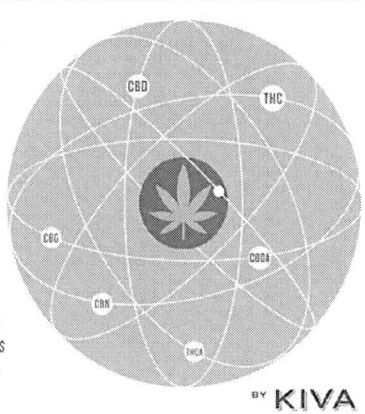

BY KIVA

This synergistic and modifying effect is known as the 'Entourage Effect'. The presence of CBD*plus*, other cannabinoids and terpenes actually has a more natural effect on the body's Endocannabinoid System (ECS).

The Entourage Effect is used in the development of cannabis-based medications, which are often presented by their ratios of CBD to THC.

For example, the best tinctures for childhood seizures have a ratio of 18:1, meaning that it is very high in CBD with only minimal amounts of THC. Pain is usually best treated with 1:1 medication.

THC

Tetrahydrocannabinol (THC) is one of the two medically important cannabinoids found in the highest levels in cannabis. THC is a psychoactive cannabinoid, as well as the component in cannabis associated with all of the significant adverse effects.

Although this may be, THC has a wide array of important medical effects that differ in many ways from CBD*plus*. As you might have guessed, THC is the cannabinoid associated with addiction.

However, when THC is combined with CBD in a 1:1 ratio, the euphoric effect caused by THC, as well as the chance of developing an addiction, is greatly reduced. THC is also associated with uncovering psychotic or paranoid behavior.

Again, using CBD in combination with the THC greatly reduces the chance of getting psychotic symptoms. In fact, pure a dose of 100-200 milligrams of a tincture or vaporizer of CBD can be given to someone having bad effects from recreational cannabis, to rapidly decrease these adverse effects.

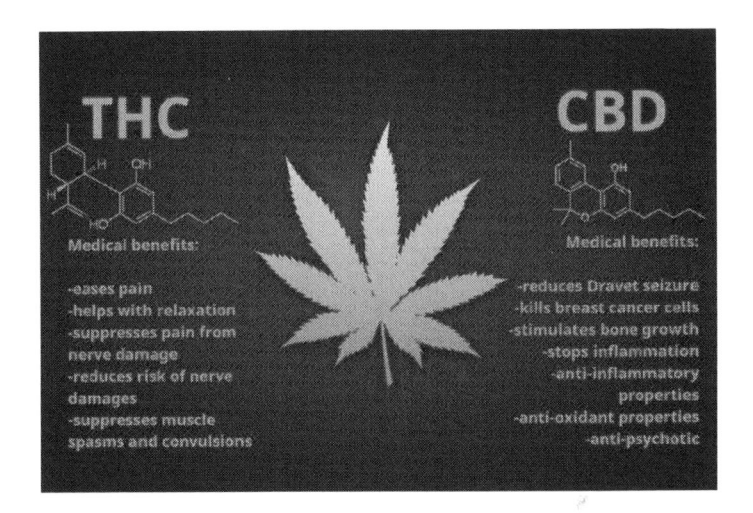

Other Cannabinoids

Since there are over 100 different cannabinoids, I am going to discuss only those that are more medically important. Additionally, the different names for each cannabinoid often sound quite similar; therefore, it is best to use the specific abbreviation that has been developed for each cannabinoid.

Every cannabinoid interacts with receptors of the body's innate Endocannabinoid System (ECS) to varying degrees and with varying health and euphoric effects. Again, because of the federal restriction on studying cannabis since 1970, there has been very little research done on these lesser cannabinoid oils.

31

CBC - cannabichromene
No euphoric effects. May have anti-inflammatory and anti-viral effects and facilitate pain relief. It also may have anti-depressant effects.

CBG – cannabigerol
No euphoric effects. May promote bone growth and have anti-inflammatory effects. Currently under study for its ability to inhibit tumor and cancer cell growth.

CBN - cannabinol
No euphoric effects. May promote bone growth and have anti-inflammatory effects. Currently under study for insomnia and inducing sleep.

11-OH-THC - eleven hydroxytetrahydrocannabinol
Intense euphoric effects. This is not present in the plant, but when the liver metabolizes THC it turns mostly into 11-OH-THC. It is considered the main active metabolite of THC after being consumed in an edible. It is more potent than THC and crosses into the brain easier than THC. It is associated with increased appetite.

Acidic Forms of Cannabinoids

All cannabinoids have an acidic carboxylated form notated by the small letter 'a' after the abbreviation, such as THCa, CBDVa and CBDa. The acidic forms are how the cannabinoids are present in the raw plant material. After decarboxylation via heat or drying of the plant material, the acidic form is turned into the oxidized form.

The acidic form usually acts entirely differently in the body from the oxidized form. For example, THCa, does not cause euphoria and preliminary research suggests that it has many medical uses different from THC.

The only way to get THCa or other acidic cannabinoids is to juice freshly harvested cannabis flowers and drink the fresh juice. If the juice is left for several days it will naturally oxidize from THCa to THC, and so on.

> For complete and up-to-date patient-oriented information on cannabinoids and terpenes go to: www.Leafly.com/news/cannabis-101

How is CBD*plus* Extracted

The oils in cannabis, including the cannabinoids and terpenes, have been extracted via various methods for over a hundred years. The extracted oils are then further processed to increase the percentage of all or specific cannabinoids.

A wide variety of solvents are used to dissolve the oils in the plant material. The type of extraction methodology will determine what contaminants are in the extract. Repeated extraction techniques result in less and less residual plant material, and consequently a lighter and clearer fluid.

Different extraction techniques can absorb different oils from the plant more or less effectively. Olive oil, and ethanol usually extract more of the terpenes than the other solvents.

Hydrocarbon Solvents

Various hydrocarbons, including benzene, butane, hexane, and propane, can be used to dissolve the oil into a liquid. A slight remnant of these solvents usually remains in the extract.

Since these hydrocarbons can contain carcinogens, especially after heating, extracts made using these solvents are not recommended.

Ingestible Solvents

Several ingestible solvents, such as ethanol, olive oil, coconut oil and butter, can be used to dissolve the cannabinoids into an edible liquid. These are safe and of course edible. However, the food grade oils, are perishable. These extracts are generally made for ingestion as an extract, or in cannabis butter for making edibles.

Carbon Dioxide

Either supercritical or subcritical carbon dioxide (CO_2) extraction, is currently the safest and most popular means of obtaining high purity extracts.

Carbon dioxide extracts an oil which very high in purity and is free from chlorophyll, and most other plant contaminants. It is used under high pressure and at extremely low temperatures to isolate the medicinal oils from the contaminants often present with other extraction methodologies. CO_2 extractions are used for an extract that is to be inhaled or ingeste

CHAPTER 2: HISTORY AND LEGAL ISSUES OF HEMP OIL USE

> *This chapter is based on a similar chapter in Dr. Smith's textbook for medical professionals, 'Medical Cannabis: Basic Science & Clinical Applications' from www.AylesburyPress.com. Several paragraphs are used directly from this textbook.*

During human evolution many plants have been discovered to have euphoric or medicinal effects. The earliest medications that our ancestors used were from plants, such as opium for pain, foxglove and digitalis for heart failure, willow bark and aspirin for pain, and cinchonine and quinine.

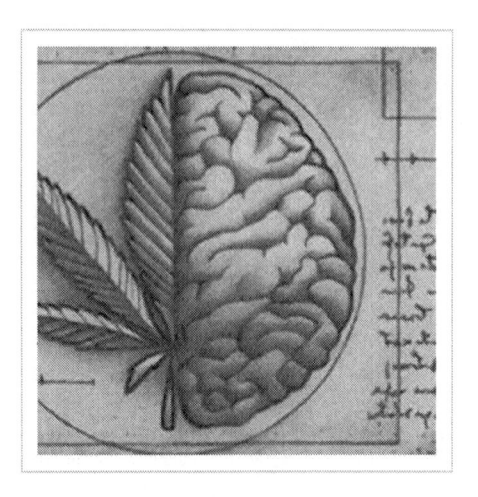

Cannabis with its often-poignant aroma and rapid onset of effects was bound to be discovered by our ancient ancestors. *Cannabis sativa* grows naturally in many tropical parts of the world and has been used for its fiber and oil-bearing seeds for 11,000

years. Cannabis plants were made into fiber for cloth and rope, and the oil from the seeds was used for a variety of household uses.

Ancient Use of Cannabis

The first recorded medical use of cannabis was described in Indo Chinese medical texts more than 5,000 years ago. At that time, it was found to be useful for a variety of both physical and mental conditions. A Chinese medical text of the time prescribed cannabis leaves for tapeworm. The seeds were pulverized and added to wine to help with constipation and hair loss.

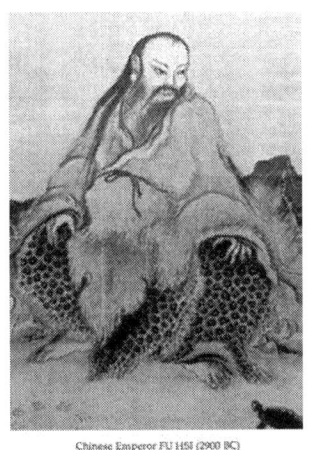

Cannabis use for recreational and medicinal effects spread throughout the Greek and Roman empires, and subsequently throughout the Islamic empire. Herodotus in 440 B.C.E. discussed the Scythians using cannabis to make a vapor for steam baths. By the Middle Ages it was regularly used externally as a balm for muscle and joint pain.

Chinese Emperor FU HSI (2900 BC) recommended medical cannabis

Cannabis was introduced to the America's by the Spaniards in 1545 for use as fiber. Hemp became the first major fiber producing plant in the U.S. By 1619 King James I ordered every colonist to grow 100 plants specifically for export. Hemp was a major crop throughout the Americas by the 18th century.

Western Medical Use of Cannabis

Although cannabis plants were ubiquitous throughout the U.S., cannabis as a medicine did not make its way into Western medicine until the 1839.

At that time, Dr. William B. O'Shaughnessy returned from India with considerable experience using cannabis for medical purposes. He encouraged physicians to recommend it for insomnia, pain, muscle spasms and other physical conditions. It soon became an accepted treatment.

After its introduction and widespread acceptance into medical practice of the time, it started to be used for a wide variety of ailments, including gonorrhea, cholera, whooping cough and asthma. It was predominantly used as an orally ingested tincture. It is said that Queen Victoria used cannabis tincture for menstrual cramps.

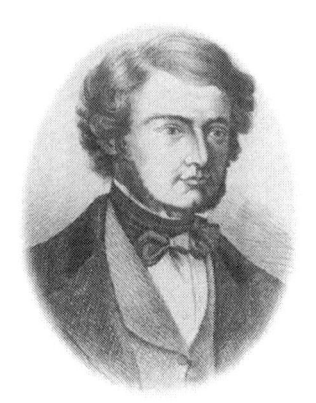

William Brooke O'Shaughnessy
1809-1889

Cannabis Indica Tincture

The potency, efficacy and side effects of various medicinal preparations of cannabis extracts varied significantly. For decades these tinctures were sold a "patent medicines" and therefore the ingredients were secret. By the late 19th century, laws were already being enacted to address issues with mislabeling, adulteration, and sale of "poisons."

Cannabis Indica Tincture

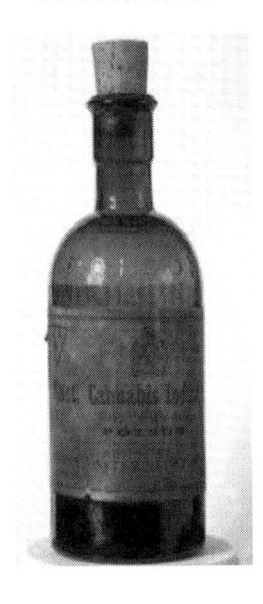

In addition, smoking cannabis for recreational use in upscale hashish parlors flourished next to the thriving opium dens of the late 19th century.

With the turn of the 20th century, laws in several states required prescriptions for cannabis extracts. By this time, cannabis was the second most common ingredient in medications and there were over 2000 cannabis containing preparations from over 280 manufacturers.

U.S. Cannabis Laws

The Pure Food and Drug Act of 1906 and several state's laws were passed to restrict "habit-forming drugs." Most of these laws were started to counteract the huge impact of heroin-use that started injured Civil War veterans with the invention of the hypodermic needles. These were the start are a series of laws to control and regulate all "euphoric" drugs.

In addition, smoking cannabis for the first time was becoming popular in the population because of over a decade of alcohol prohibition. This lead to a backlash against smoking cannabis, which was previously acceptable only among Mexican migrant workers and Negro Jazz musicians. The term "marihuana"—later changed to cannabis—was a slang term used by Mexican immigrants to describe cannabis, meaning "Mary Jane" in Spanish.

The federal government began use the term cannabis in all government documents to separate 'smoked' cannabis from the very popular *cannabis sativa* elixirs that were used medicinally. The movie "Reefer Madness" (1938) is a classic example of this hysteria of this era. At the same time, the Cannabis Tax Act of 1937 imposed a levy of one dollar per ounce on cannabis used for medical use and $100 per ounce for recreational use. This law effectively made non-medical or non-industrial use, possession or sale of cannabis illegal throughout the U.S. At that time, the fledgling American Medical Association (A.M.A.) was against this law, and correctly thought that it would impede future research into the drug.

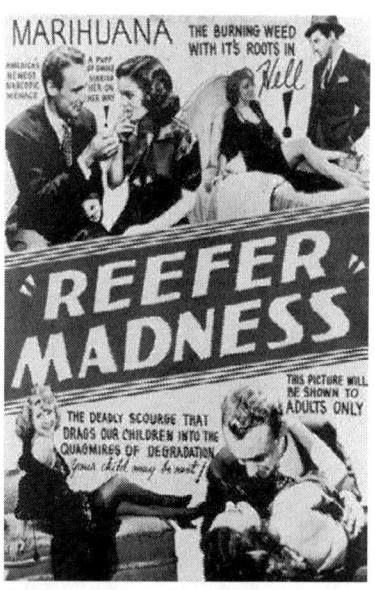

By 1938, the Federal Pure Food, Drug and Cosmetics Act established the framework that we still use today to regulate prescription and non-prescriptions drugs. By 1951, the Boggs Act, added *cannabis sativa* to the list of narcotic drugs. The use of cannabis for medical purposes dramatically decreased over the course of the early twentieth century. There was some research in the 50's and 60's for use in glaucoma. But far superior ophthalmic medications were soon to become available.

THC was not isolated from *cannabis sativa* until Dr. Raphael Mechoulam discovered it in Israel in

1964. THCV (CBDplus) had been isolated several years earlier, along with dozens of other cannabinoids. In the 70's, a synthetic version of THC called Marinol® was approved for chemotherapy induced nausea and vomiting, and later for cancer and AIDS-related wasting syndrome. However, the intense euphoric side effects from pure THC and need to swallow oral capsules while feeling nauseous made this a poor clinical choice. The advent of superior medications had practically deemed the use of synthetic THC pharmaceuticals obsolete.

In 1969, during a very turbulent period of "anti-war" social unrest, president Nixon pushed for a comprehensive restructuring of drug laws, for what he called the "war on drugs." He was especially focused on cannabis because of its association with the "anti-war" movement. The Controlled Substances Act (C.S.A.) was passed as part of the Comprehensive Drug Abuse Prevention and Control Act of 1970. This made the possession or distribution of *cannabis sativa* a criminal offense under federal law. This legislation created the five Schedules of Dangerous Drugs, and The Drug Enforcement Administration (D.E.A.) and Food and Drug Administration (F.D.A.) were both to determine which drugs are placed into the Schedules. It placed cannabis into Schedule I, where the drug was determined to have no medical use and had a high risk of addiction.

> See the following website for the current status of cannabis, CBD, THC and THCV (CBD*plus*) laws in the US.
>
> www.wikipedia.org/wiki/Legality of cannabis by U. S. jurisdiction

CBD*plus* Research

This legislation effectively put an end to all serious scientific study of medical cannabis, including THC, CBD and CBD*plus*, and also severely limited the study of the cannabinoids. In the early 1990's, the Endocannabinoid System (ECS) was discovered, and we learned that cannabinoids effect the body by binding to natural cannabinoid receptors in the brain and body that make up the ECS.

Since this natural system in our body was discovered, researchers have conducted tens of thousands of studies in animal models and tissue culture on the effects of the various cannabinoids; however, the main research on CBD, CBD*plus*, and CBDV in humans has been done in trials by GW Pharmaceuticals. CBD is one of the three cannabinoids present in high quantities in cannabis and a growing body of research has shown how CBD*plus* can also have a wide array of beneficial medical effects.

U.S. Medical Cannabis Laws

In 1996, after several failed attempts, California was the first state to pass Proposition 215—also known as the Compassionate Care Act. This Act, along with Senate Bill 420 in 2003, allowed for a network of growers, caregivers, healthcare providers, and an identification card system for medical cannabis. At the time these laws were written, 42 states and the District of Columbia have some sort of legalized medical cannabis laws.

Whole Plant Versus CBD or THCV Only Laws

Whole-plant cannabis refers to having measurable quantities of THC, so that there may be euphoric effects. Many of the states allow for CBD and CBD*plus* only; meaning, that the plant or extract has very low amounts of THC and high amounts of CBD and/or CBD*plus*. Charlotte's Web is an example of a cannabis strain that is very low in THC and high in CBD. Most of the laws that allow for CBD only state that this medicine can be used to treat intractable seizures only.

Some countries have taken a much more practical approach to defining medical cannabis. In these countries, as long as the ratio of CBD to THC is 1:1 or greater (higher in CBD) then it is considered legal for medical use. This is a wise approach as CBD significantly decreases the euphoric effects of THC, and CBD blocks almost all of the adverse side effects—such as paranoia, anxiety, agitation and addiction—that come from THC. Furthermore, it is very important to note that it is highly unusual and unlikely for a patient to become addicted or dependent from the use of high CBD or CBD*plus* medical cannabis.

When it comes to regulations and requirements of CBD and CBD*plus*, it is essential to know that they vary considerably among states in the U.S. and countries around the globe. For example, New York allows for medical cannabis as long as it isn't smoked. Some territories allow for the use of medical cannabis only for Qualified Conditions (QC), such as Multiple Sclerosis or Alzheimer's disease.

The QC's vary considerably from state to state and are based on political and not scientific motives. That being said, it is the efficacy of THC, CBD and CBDplus as well as their innate safety, that has been generally recognized as the underpinnings to support and continue the expansion of medical cannabis laws in the U.S. and around the world.

Changes in Federal Cannabis Policy

In 2009—based on the rapidly evolving changes at the state level in legalization of medical cannabis—the U.S. Attorney General stated, "It will not be a priority to use federal resources to prosecute patients with serious illnesses or their caregivers who are complying with state laws on medical cannabis, but we will not tolerate drug traffickers who hide behind claims of compliance with state law to mask activities that are clearly illegal."

In December 2014, congress and the Obama administration quietly put an end to the federal prohibition against medical cannabis as a tiny part of a federal spending bill. However, federal banking laws still force medical dispensaries to operate as "cash only" businesses. Most recently, the prescription opioid epidemic that has been ravaging the U.S., has helped push cannabis into the spotlight as a much safer and less toxic alternative to opioids for pain control. Cannabis has been shown to be very helpful with transitioning patients off opioids.

Although the F.D.A. continues to have *cannabis sativa* as a Schedule I drug, there are major efforts underway to reschedule to a lower schedule drug classification, or to perhaps de-schedule cannabis as a medicine to be treated like alcohol or tobacco regulated substances instead.

CBD*plus* Laws in the United States

Non-hemp *cannabis sativa*, as well as any extracts from the cannabis plant, are still considered an illegal drug at the federal level in the U.S., and therefore require a doctor's recommendation letter within the 29 states where it is legal. Even extracts of pure CBD*plus*, if they originated in the flower of the non-hemp *cannabis sativa* plant, are considered illegal drugs. Only CBD*plus* oil that originates in legal hemp plants is considered legal by law and is available online and in all 50 states.

On February 7, 2014, President Obama signed the Farm Bill of 2013 into law, and section 7606 of the act—the Legitimacy of Industrial Hemp Research—defines industrial hemp as entirely distinct from cannabis, and authorizes—for the first time in the U.S. since 1937—for institutions of higher education and state departments of agriculture (in states where hemp cultivation is legalized) to regulate and conduct research and pilot programs. So far, 31 states have defined industrial hemp as distinct from cannabis and have removed barriers to it production. This has led to a plethora of high quality, U.S. grown hemp oil to become available.

To further support the intent of the 2014 Farm Bill and to stop efforts of the DEA to control CBD*plus* and the expanding state medical cannabis laws, the Appropriations Act of 2017, Sec 773, explicitly states that federal funds may not be used to:

> "prohibit the transportation, processing, sale, or use of industrial hemp that is grown or cultivated in accordance with section 7606 of the Agricultural Act of 2014, within or outside the State in which the industrial hemp is grown or cultivated."

Therefore, legal and over-the-counter CBD*plus* products are manufactured from legally cultivated hemp and are exactly the same as CBD*plus* from other sources. The upcoming Farm Bill of 2018 will supposedly further clarify the legality of hemp oil derivatives such as CBD and CBD*plus*.

CBD*plus* Laws in Other Countries

Pure CBD, CBD*plus* or low-THC hemp oil is typically not considered a scheduled substance or an illegal drug anywhere in the world; however, it is generally considered to be a hemp oil, a cosmetic ingredient or a nutritional supplement.

Although it is considered to be a controlled substance in some countries and requires a prescription from a physician, the World Health Organization recommended that CBD no longer be listed as a controlled substance in 2017.

Epididolex®

A pharmaceutical company out of the U.K. has been developing several cannabis-based prescription medications over the past 20 years. One of these medications, called Epidiolex®, is 99% CBD extracted from the flowers of a specific strain of *cannabis sativa*. It has recently been given and "orphan drug designation" by the FDA for the treatment of two very rare forms of childhood intractable seizures. This means that this drug may very soon become available by prescription in the U.S. for these conditions. It will probably cost $18,000-$30,000 a year for this prescription medication, unlike other better whole-plant CBD extracts that are readily available online or in stores for around $1200 a year.

The recent FDA recognition of this 99% pure CBD as an Investigational New Drug may result in it becoming a prescription medication. This has created great concern among the many of the manufacturers of other high concentration CBD extracts that sell their products. They may have to stop selling or producing their products if this is causing patent infringement or other legal issues with the manufacturers of Epidiolex®. This is a very recent development at this time. Readers can Google Epidiolex® to learn more.

Physician Education and Cannabinoids

In 2018, it is estimated that about 1-2% of physicians in the U.S. regularly recommend medical cannabis in their practice. About 5% have had any education on the Endocannabinoid System (ECS) or training on the use of cannabinoids such as THC, CBD and *CBDplus* oils. There are several reasons for this. Even though cannabis has a long and respected history as a medicine, it was not until the early 1990's that the ECS was discovered and researchers could start to evaluate how cannabinoids work in the brain and body. So, most of today's practicing physicians were already out of medical school while the ECS was first being discovered and researched. Expectedly so, there is essentially no consistent training or education for medical students, to this day, on the science of cannabinoids, medical cannabis or the ECS.

The first medical cannabis law passed in California in 1996 and the perception of the medical community has been that medical cannabis laws were ways for people to bypass the prohibition against the recreational use of cannabis. Indeed, in many states there is strong evidence to suggest that medical cannabis laws are facilitating recreational users getting easy access to relatively inexpensive cannabis.

Eventually, *cannabis sativa* was put into Schedule I of the federal Controlled Substances Act in 1970. This federal law described cannabis as having no medical benefits and being highly addictive. Remaining as a Schedule I drug severely limited the amount of human research conducted on cannabinoids over the past 40 years. Almost all of the research done on humans is either very old, from the 70s and 80s, small poor-quality studies, or were done using synthetic pharmaceuticals and not whole-plant cannabis. Just in the past few years have high quality, whole-plant cannabis studies in humans started to be published.

In 2016, I wrote my textbook, *Medical Cannabis: Basic Science and Clinical Applications* (http://www.aylesburypress.com), because there was no science-based text available to educate medical students, physicians and other medical professionals on medical cannabis. There will probably be five different cannabinoid medications available at pharmacies around the U.S. by the end of 2018, and still this situation with physician and pharmacist training is not changing very rapidly.

CHAPTER 3: HOW DOES CBDPLUS WORK?

CBD*plus* is very safe and effective with few adverse effects. It has many medical effects in the brain and body and works on several medical conditions. Unlike THC, there is no euphoria associated with using CBD*plus* and no concern about addiction or dependency.

In general, CBD*plus* can be considered an adjunct, or helper, to be used in conjunction with other medications, dietary changes and a regular exercise regimen, that are already available. In the future, CBD*plus* may be considered preventive medicine and be taken in small, once-a-day doses to prevent or slow the progress of a wide array of common metabolic conditions.

Endocannabinoid System (ECS)

Like CBD, THC and the other minor cannabinoids, CBD*plus* works by impacting the body's Endocannabinoid System (ECS) in several different ways. The ECS is a natural system in our brain and body. It is a system that is present in all animals and fish, and evolutionarily dates back 600 million years. The ECS's job is to modulate other systems in the body that can become overheated.

It is like a braking system, that can slow down a wide variety of systems in the body, including pain perception, gastrointestinal motility, memory, sleep, response to stress, pain and appetite—just to name a few. The ECS has unique functions throughout the body, but especially within the brain and the immune system. In fact, ECS receptors are the most common receptors in the brain and the second most common receptors in the body, showing just how important the ECS is. Among the manifold roles of the ECS is the regulation of metabolism and energy expenditure.

THE ENDOCANNABINOID SYSTEM

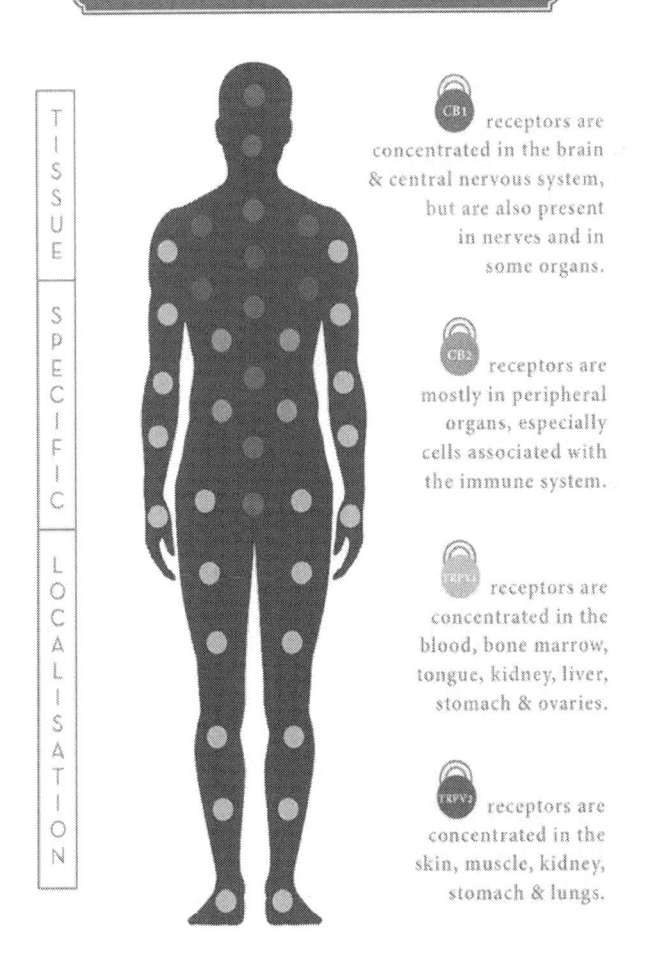

TISSUE SPECIFIC LOCALISATION

CB1 receptors are concentrated in the brain & central nervous system, but are also present in nerves and in some organs.

CB2 receptors are mostly in peripheral organs, especially cells associated with the immune system.

TRPV1 receptors are concentrated in the blood, bone marrow, tongue, kidney, liver, stomach & ovaries.

TRPV2 receptors are concentrated in the skin, muscle, kidney, stomach & lungs.

HUMAN CANNABINOID RECEPTORS

Nerve cells—called neurons—release chemical messengers called neurotransmitters. There are literally hundreds of different neurotransmitters released in the body depending on what system is involved. When there are too many chemical messengers being released and a specific system is growing out of control, the ECS releases its own specific chemical messengers on demand to slow down the release of these chemical messengers.

Thus, the ECS keeps several of the body's system in balance. The ECS uses two different chemicals, anandamide (ANA) and 2 arachidonoylglycerol (2-AG.) These chemicals are known as endocannabinoids and are the innate cannabinoids made naturally by the body. These endocannabinoids work by attaching to a cannabinoid receptor on the cell. THC and CBD*plus* work by imitating the body's naturally occurring endocannabinoids.

The two substances made by our body to unlock and activate the ECS are:

2-AG

ANA

Cannabinoids from hemp, like CBD*plus* and CBD mimic these two substances.

Endocannabinoid Receptors

There are two ECS receptors that we know of—simply named, cannabinoid receptor 1 (CB1) and cannabinoid receptor 2 (CB2.) There are possibly a few more receptors, but they have yet to be discovered. Some systems in our brain and body only have CB1 receptors while some only have CB2; and some systems have both.

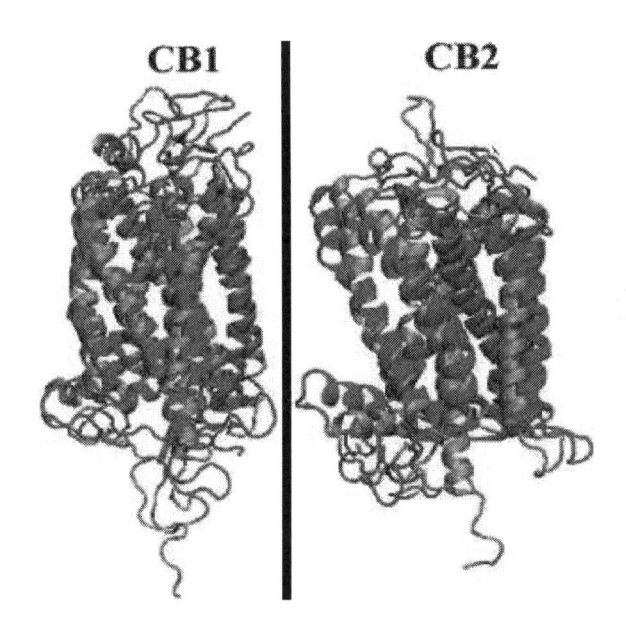

CB1 | **CB2**

Much like a lock that needs a key to open, the cannabinoid receptor on the cell membrane is the lock, while and the endocannabinoid chemical, ANA or 2-AG, is the key. Once the endocannabinoid is released it "unlocks" the receptor, which is then quickly broken down by the enzymes in the area so that, when the endocannabinoids are released in response to "stress", the effect is only short-lived—maybe milliseconds. Cannabinoids including CBD, THC and CBD*plus* do not have local enzymes to break them down once they unlock a receptor, and therefore last a long time as they remain in the unlocked receptor to provide therapeutic effects for many hours after each dose.

Once inhaled or ingested, plant-based cannabinoids including CBD, CBD*plus* and THC present in the hemp oil get into the bloodstream and travel all over the brain and body. These cannabinoids then bind to CB1 and CB2 receptors in the brain and certain organs in the body just as ANA and 2-AG do. This results in similar effects to the body's endocannabinoid chemicals, 2-AG and ANA. When we use hemp oil, however, it can have a much greater impact on our body's ECS when compared to ANA and 2-AG alone; thus producing both medical and therapeutic effects. Since there are no specific enzymes in the body to immediately break down these hemp oils, these effects last much longer.

The following graphic is from www.Canna-pet.com. It shows how CBD works with the ECS.

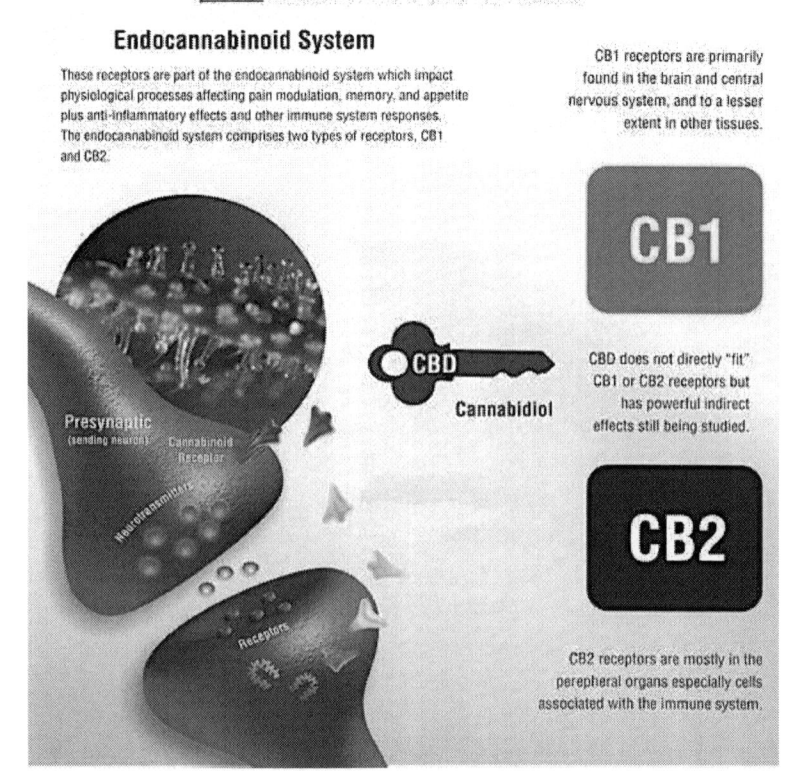

Endocannabinoid System

These receptors are part of the endocannabinoid system which impact physiological processes affecting pain modulation, memory, and appetite plus anti-inflammatory effects and other immune system responses. The endocannabinoid system comprises two types of receptors, CB1 and CB2.

CB1 receptors are primarily found in the brain and central nervous system, and to a lesser extent in other tissues.

CB1

CBD does not directly "fit" CB1 or CB2 receptors but has powerful indirect effects still being studied.

Cannabidiol

CB2

CB2 receptors are mostly in the peripheral organs especially cells associated with the immune system.

Different cannabinoids in cannabis interact directly or indirectly with the CB1 and CB2 receptors. The way in which the cannabinoids interact with these receptors, determines what medical effects and what adverse side effects we can expect.

CBD*plus* directly interacts with both the CB1 or CB2 receptors and also physically blocks the receptor so that ANA, 2-AG or THC cannot attach to the receptor to stimulate it. In essence, CBD*plus* has the exact opposite effects of THC in the brain. In the body, CBD*plus* stimulates CB2 receptors and has many actions similar therapeutic effects similar to CBD. Because of this, CBD and CBD*plus* can work well together to have a combined effect at the CB1 (brain) and CB2 (immune system) cells.

CB1 Receptors

The CB1 receptors are mostly found in certain brain centers. Here is a list of most of the brain centers and their associated function:

Hippocampus - Learning, memory, stress related to adverse memories

Hypothalamus- Appetite

Limbic System- Anxiety

Cerebral Cortex- Pain processing, higher cognitive functions

Nucleus Accumbens-   Reward and Addiction

Basal Ganglia- Sleep, movement

Medulla- Nausea and vomiting chemoreceptor

There are quite a few organs in the body that also have CB1 receptors as well, including the uterus, cardiovascular system, adipose tissue, gastrointestinal tract, pancreas, bone and liver. We are still learning exactly how the ECS modulates these organs. By blocking our naturally occurring endocannabinoids, CBD*plus* has very interesting and novel therapeutic effects such as the "anti-munchies".

At the low doses of CBD*plus* recommended throughout this book—less than 20mg per dose—CBD*plus* functions by blocking the CB1 receptor. At high doses, it can actually start stimulating the CB1 receptor and may result in some euphoric effects similar to THC. However, this is not a concern at the doses of CBD*plus* recommended throughout this book.

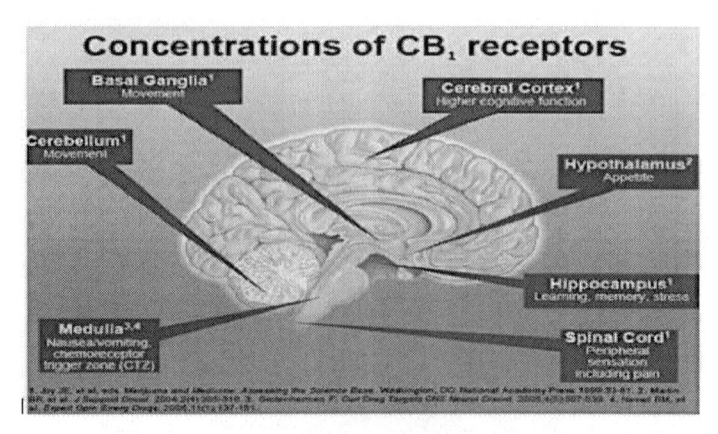

The above graphic, from theleafonline.com shows CB1 receptors in the brain.

CB2 Receptors

The CB2 receptors are found mostly in the immune system cells in the brain and body. These cells are involved with immunity and inflammation, and with CB2 receptors, include monocytes, macrophages, B-cells, T-cells, and thymus gland cells—all of which have to do with modulating the release of chemicals involved with swelling, immune response, cell migration and programmed cell death. In general, when the receptors are activated the immune or inflammatory response is turned down.

CB2 receptors are also found in our bone's osteoblast cells. These cells work in tandem with osteoclasts to create new healthy bone cells. Studies have shown that activation of CB2 receptors results in improved healing of fractures. Many tissues or organs of the body have both CB1 and CB2 receptors, providing different, often counter-balancing functions. Some of these include: skin, brain, liver, and bone.

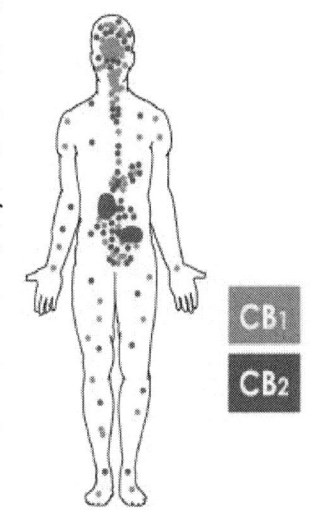

CBD*plus* stimulates CB2 receptors, as do CBD and cannabidivarin (CBDV). So, it has many of the same positive therapeutic effects on inflammation, pain, irritable bowel syndrome, and other CB2 receptor mediated medical effects.

Change in Number of Receptors

The number or density of these ECS receptors, shaped like little buttons in the membrane of a cell, is determined by how easily the receptors are activated. If there is excess of stimulation of these receptors over time, then the number of receptors on the cell membrane will tend to decrease. This is called 'down-regulation'.

Because of this, it will take more of the cannabinoid to get the same effect. If there is not enough stimulation of these receptors, the number of receptors will tend to increase over time. This is called 'up-regulation' and will result in more effects from lower doses of cannabinoids.

In order to learn how to dose CBD*plus* effectively, it is important to understand the importance of finding just the right dose that does not result in up- or down-regulation of the receptors on the cell membranes.

THC

When THC binds to the receptors, it only partially opens the lock. This is called being a 'partial stimulator'. THC binds to both CB1 and CB2 receptors, and the euphoric effects of THC are due to the CB1 binding in certain brain centers. THC is one of the few well studied cannabinoids that has consistent binding on CB1 receptors.

CBD*plus* (THCV)

CBD*plus* works via the ECS. It physically blocks the CB1 receptors—mostly in the brain—which prevents the body's natural endocannabinoids and THC from working. This results in decreased appetite and has positive effects of nausea and vomiting. CBD*plus* also activates CB2 receptors—mostly on the immune system cells—and decreases degenerative changes in the immune system, some types of pain, as well as inflammation. CBD*plus* has been shown to have beneficial effects on seizures, similar to CBD. Anecdotal evidence in humans and studies in animal models suggests adding CBD*plus* to CBD to get improved control of seizures.

CBDV

CBDV has many similarities to CBD*plus*. Most importantly it does not cause euphoria, and it works similarly to CBD*plus* to decrease appetite, and decreased nausea and vomiting. CBD*plus* has been shown to have beneficial effects on seizures similar to CBD as well. Anecdotal evidence in humans and studies in animal models suggests adding CBDV to CBD to get improved control of seizures.

Other Effects

The vast majority of the medical effects of cannabis occur by impacting the ECS. However, the various cannabinoid oils have other beneficial therapeutic effects that don't necessarily work through the ECS. Cannabinoids are potent antioxidants and can have effects by counteracting the adverse effects of oxidative stress. In addition, THC has been shown to block the effects of certain enzymes and have beneficial effects in this way as well.

Using Hemp Oil Medications

There are many ways to get cannabinoid medication into the body. The ways in which the cannabinoid journeys into the bloodstream, from the blood stream to the brain, and throughout the rest of the body is very important. The four main methods of taking cannabis medications include inhalation, ingestion, mucous membrane absorption and topical application.

Inhalation

Inhaling implies smoking or vaporizing bud, hashish or oil. When the material is smoked, it is actually combusted, and many products of combustion go along with the vaporized oil into the lungs. Smoking cannabis results in incineration of half of the bud, so that only half of oils make into the inhalation into the lungs.

Only about 10% of the "smoke" is actually the therapeutic oils. The remaining 90% is a merely a hodgepodge of potentially carcinogenic hydrocarbons and inert plant particulates. However, several good studies have failed to find an association with long term smoking of cannabis and increased rates of respiratory tract cancer. It is felt that the anti-cancer effects of THC, and CBD probably cancel out the adverse effects of the carcinogens. However, this matter has not been clearly settled with high quality studies.

When the bud, hashish or oil is heated to a certain temperature (usually around 320-360 degrees Fahrenheit) there is no combustion; there is only vaporization of the cannabinoids and terpenes along with a very small quantity of potentially carcinogenic hydrocarbons present in the plant material. Vaporizing is much more effective, considering that as much as 90% of the THC and CBD*plus* oils reach the lungs upon inhaling.

Inhalation leads to direct and rapid entry into the bloodstream via the lungs. It results in effective concentrations of cannabinoids in the bloodstream within a few minutes and maximum effect within 15 minutes. However, beneficial effects only last 45-60 minutes. Because of its rapid entrance into the body, inhalation is good for immediate relief of pain, inflammation or spasm. An inhaled dose usually starts having effects within minutes and usually lasts about one to one and a half hours.

Ingestion

Ingestion implies eating, drinking or swallowing droplets of a tincture or an extract into the mouth and swallowing it so that it goes into the stomach. It is then absorbed in the duodenum and goes through the liver before ever getting in the blood stream. While in the liver the oils are metabolized by a series of enzymes, making much of the original CBD or CBD*plus* unusable. These medications for ingestion are usually extracted with coconut or olive made into an extract or with alcohol and made into a tincture. There are also infused drinks, cooked or baked edibles. This process is much slower, with the onset of action taking 1 ½ to 2 hours from ingestion. This slow onset is known as the 'first-pass effect' and is a phase that you may hear often. It refers to the fact that when a medication is swallowed it goes into the intestine and is passed through the liver. In the liver the CBD and THC are metabolized to different chemicals, THC is metabolized to 11-OH-THC, and CBD to 7-OH-CBD and CBD-7-oic acid. The end result for CBD is that only about 15% of it is available after it goes through the liver, the rest has been broken down into inactive metabolites. Also, 90% of the THC is metabolized into other chemicals via the 'first pass effect". In the case of THC, it is metabolized into 11-OH-THC. 11-OH-THC is actually a much more potent than regular THC.

There has been very little research on the metabolism of CBD*plus*. In general, it should be considered to be metabolized the same way as CBD, so that oromusocal (under the tongue) absorption or inhalation (vaporizing) are the preferred ways to take it as a medicine. Much of the CBD*plus* will be broken down into inactive metabolites if it is ingested (eaten, swallowed) and allowed to go through the 'first pass effect.' So, the effects of ingested vs. inhaled cannabis medication can be quite different.

Mucous Membrane Absorption

There are several preparations of cannabinoid medications that are meant to be absorbed via a mucous membrane, the nose, the mouth cavity, or the rectum. For the nose and mouth, it is usually in the form of a spray or mist that is inhaled through the nose or sprayed inside the mouth, a mouth strip (similar to a breath strip) or an extract. For the rectum, it is usually a rectal suppository. When cannabinoid medication is meant to be taken in this way, it is usually absorbed into the bloodstream through local absorption through thin and very vascular mucous membranes. Thus, absorbed medications tend to work more quickly compared to when ingested, and tend to work longer than inhaled medications as well. Much faster than edibles, they are absorbed within 30 minutes; but they only last 2-3 hours, which is shorter than edibles. However, there is no 'first-pass effect', so they are not broken down into metabolites right away like edibles are.

Extracts and tinctures can function as two different medications: slow release or fast release. If the extract is placed on the tongue (see photograph I) and then swished around the front of the mouth with the tongue (see photograph II), then it will absorb rapidly and miss the 'first-pass effect.' This results in rapid onset of symptom relief that lasts 1-2 hours. If the same extract is swallowed immediately, or put in a tea and ingested, then it will go through the 'first-pass effect' and both absorb more slowly and last much longer.

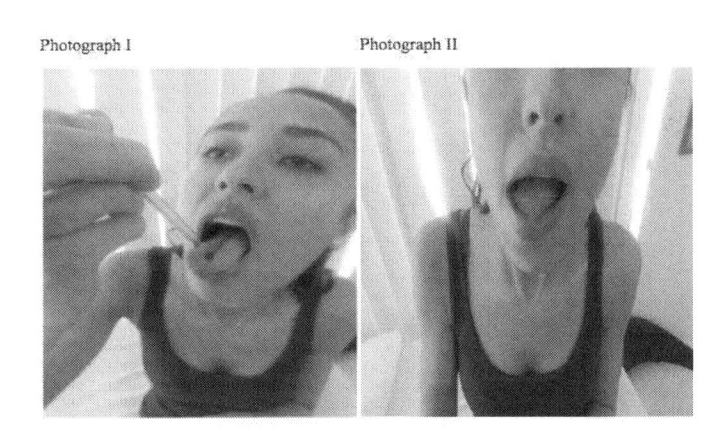

Photograph I   Photograph II

Applying to the Skin

Topical application of cannabinoid medications can work in one of two ways: as a salve or as a slow-release patch or gel. As a salve, they are absorbed only locally by painful or inflamed tissues.

63

For example, salve can be applied to the area of a painful arthritic joint or inflamed skin conditions. Often these salves are combined with other active ingredients like camphor, menthol and capsaicin which also have local effects on pain and inflammation.

Another way in which topical cannabinoid medication works is in the form of a patch or gel which is meant to result is a constant slow absorption of cannabinoids through the skin and into the bloodstream. These topical cannabinoids have a very slow onset of action and result in a constant low level of cannabinoids medications for up to 24 hours with one application. However, the absorption is highly variable from person to person.

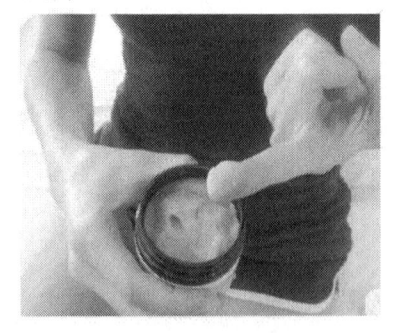

Photograph III

Photograph IV

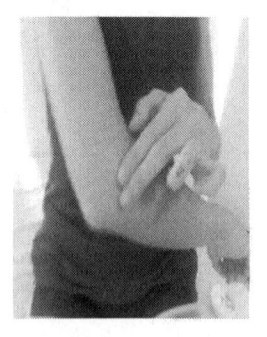

There are plenty of CB1 and CB2 receptors in the skin, in the tissues immediately under the skin, and around joints of the hands, feet, elbows, knees, and shoulders that can will absorb CBD*plus* that are applied topically over a local area. Use a small amount around the size of a dime (see photograph III), rub it in with deep pressure and leave a thin layer over the inflamed skin or joint (see photograph IV).

Forms of the Medication

It is important to have a working knowledge of how the medication can be purchased for use online, at a store, or without a prescription in all 50 states. As was discussed previously, legal hemp oil products must originate from hemp (less than 0.3% THC) grown either outside of the U.S., or legally inside of the U.S. under the 2014 Farm Bill. Therefore, if you are in a state where medical cannabis—in this case, CBD*plus*—is legal, it can come from any source— either hemp or cannabis plants.

> There are several websites that may be useful to find legal CBD*plus* either at a nearby location, or for online purchase. Here are a few
>
> http://www.TheHempDepot.org
>
> www.CBDoilreviews.com
>
> www.CWhemp.com

Flowering Bud

In general, *cannabis sativa* bud that is high in CBD*plus* and has less than 0.3% THC will only be available to purchase in a dispensary in states that have medical or recreational cannabis laws. It is typically not legal to get high THCV/low THC bud online or in non-legal states. In non-legal states, extracts, tinctures, mouth strips, various types of edibles and vaporizers are usually available in stores or online.

Even with the dozens of other means of ingesting cannabis, smoking is still by far the most common—even for medical use. I believe that everyone should be familiar with the fat, green 'bud' that is associated with cannabis. Different strains of cannabis have been bred over the decades that have focused on maximizing the percentage of THC and/or CBD*plus* in the bud.

There are literally hundreds of different strains of cannabis, with new ones being genetically engineered regularly. Many strains are often named after the aromas given off by the terpenes in the bud, or by the color of the cannabis resin glands called trichomes. Some examples of high CBD*plus*/low THC strains were discussed in a 2014 article of High Times magazine. It is important to note that a strain high in CBD*plus* may only be 1-2% THCV. There are no very highly concentrated strains, such as 10-30%, at this time.

High Times Article

Tangie, a cross of Cali Orange and a Skunk hybrid, has a modest 0.3 % THCV (CBD*plus*) due to its skunky origins. Pie Face OG, a cross of Cherry Pie and "Face Off" OG Kush, has almost 0.5 % THCV because of its Durban Poison genes: Cherry Pie is a cross of Grand Daddy Purple and Durban Poison. <u>Girl Scout Cookies</u> also has some THCV (CBD*plus*) from its Durban Poison origins, but not in any significant quantity. Hawaiian Dutch (Dutch #5 Female x Sweet Hawaiian) has almost 0.5 % THCV (CBD*plus*), likely because of its Dutch lineage.
The highest-testing flower for THCV (CBD*plus*) at the 2014 High Times Seattle U.S. Cannabis Cup was Durban Poison by TJ'S Organic Gardens, which took third place in the

U.S. *Sativa* category. THCV (CBD*plus*) was almost 1 % of the flowers' total mass.

The concentrate that tested the highest for THCV (CBD*plus*) at that same cup was Ace of Spades Shatter by Category 5 Research. This cross of Jack the Ripper and Black Cherry Soda had 2.4 % THCV (CBD*plus*), but it didn't win any awards in the U.S. Concentrates category. Agent Orange Nug Run Shatter (Agent Orange x Jack the Ripper) by A Greener Today North took Fifth Place in the Medical Concentrate category and had almost 2 % THCV (CBD*plus*).

Most people reading this book will be buying extracts or vaporizers that contain high concentrations of CBD*plus* that have been extracted from a high-CBD*plus* strain of cannabis.

The different strains of cannabis at a dispensary will often have a label stating the concentrations of THC, CBD, and sometimes THCV (CBD*plus*). Remember, that the real scientific term for CBD*plus* is THCV, and this is the term that will be used on labels and official scientific documents. The clinician and patient should be aware that these labels are notoriously inaccurate. Each new batch of bud may have markedly different potency, even if it came from the same dispensary and has the same name of strain. Stick the

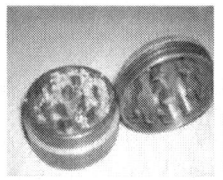

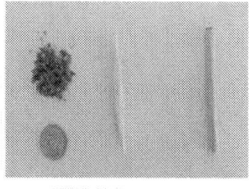

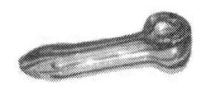

Photograph V   Photograph VI   Photograph VII

therapeutic goal of starting out with a low dose and titrate slowly up to clinical effect.

The bud is usually ground in a handheld grinder (see Photograph V) and is available at dispensaries for only a few dollars. Grinding the bud into small particles make it smoke more evenly and smoothly. When the bud is heated up by a vaporizer or burned the crystallized oil releases a fume or vapor of medication that is inhaled. The ground bud can then be smoked in rolling paper. The average joint has approximately 400-500mg of dried ground bud in it (see Photograph VI).

There are a myriad of glass and metal pipes, and water pipes, that are available (see Photograph VII). These hold large amounts of ground cannabis bud and are not generally good for use for medication purposes. There are large tabletop or large handheld vaporizers that can cost hundreds of dollars. These allow for strict control of the temperature so that the oils are aromatized at exactly the correct temperature. There are small pen vaporizers, similar to e-cigarettes (see Photograph VIII). Disposable cartridges are available containing exact amounts of CBD*plus* or whole-plant extract. Generally, each inhalation of a pen vaporizer will provide 2.0 – 2.5mg of CBD*plus*.

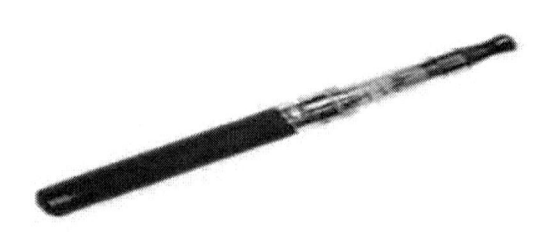

Photograph VIII

These devices vaporize CBD*plus* or whole plant (THC and CBD*plus*) oil that has been diluted in glycerin or propylene glycol. Propylene glycol is not recommended as a diluent because of health risks associated with it when it is heated. CBD*plus* oil boils at 160-180 degrees Celsius (320-356 Fahrenheit) and turns into a vapor, whereas THC oil boils at 220 Celsius (428 Fahrenheit). A joint, however, can reach 2000 degrees Fahrenheit incinerating at least half of the oil in the bud, before releasing any of the oils for inhalation.

Micro-dose Inhaler (MDI)®

More recently, the CannaKit® was created with a patented micro-dose inhaler (MDI®). The MDI® has the appearance of a cigarette (see Photograph IX) but it is actually a patented metal tube, the tip of which holds exactly 50mg of ground bud.

This allows for precise dosing of cannabis medication from 0.5mg to 6.0mg of inhaled medication. It also dramatically reduces the amount of expensive bud that is often wasted with other means of smoking. It comes with an odor-proof carrying case, which carries a couple days of ground bud, and a cleaning tool.

Visit www.CannaKitBox.com to learn more.

The clinical effects of the medication are directly related to the amount of fume that the patient inhales. The patient holds the inhaled fume in the lungs for 2-3 seconds to maximize absorption of the medication from the fume in the lungs. The patient is usually advised to start with a small, deep inhalation of the fume. When there is THC in the bud, the initial effect of the medication is usually some euphoria which can start within a couple of minutes after the initial dose.

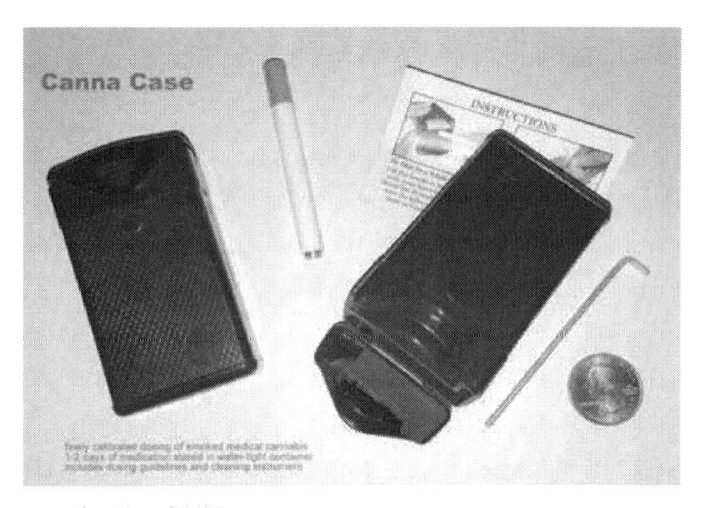

Photograph IX

Since CBD*plus* has no euphoric effects, there are no obvious sensations or effects initially. CBD*plus* reaches a peak dose in the blood after about 9-23 minutes and it is at this time that the relaxing, anti-anxiety effects become noticeable. Because the medication is inhaled and bypasses the liver first-pass effect that occurs with eating or swallowing the medications, it starts working much more quickly but last a much shorter duration of one to one and a half hours.

Smoking or vaporizing cannabis is most useful for episodic need for the medication for acute flare-ups of pain, spasms, seizures, and anxiety. Smoking bud for medical purposes has several pitfalls. The first pitfall is the obvious and often intense lingering aroma that is associated with the exhaled smoke. Since cannabis is still considered an illegal drug when used for non-medical purposes in many places, it can oftentimes lead to legal and social issues. The second pitfall is that the cannabis smoke is made up of hundreds of by-products; some of which are known respiratory tract irritants. Because of this, clinicians wouldn't want to recommend use of smoked bud in patients with certain respiratory tract conditions, or for use in and around children or people with respiratory tracts conditions.

It is important to note, however, that the smoke-related by-products have not been associated with increased rates of respiratory tract cancer. Also, vaporizing the bud at lower temperatures (instead of igniting the bud when smoking it) releases much higher concentrations of the pure medicine, and markedly less by-products.

Hashish

Hashish is made from the compressed resin glands of the cannabis bud. It contains all of the same active ingredients as the bud but is more concentrated. The exact hardness of the hashish varies significantly and depends on how it is prepared.

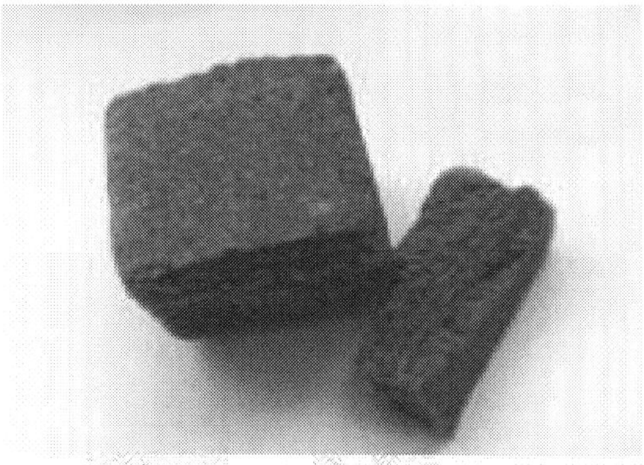

Photograph X

It can be hard and waxy, soft and pasty or come as an oil. The color ranges from earthy browns, to tan and yellowish red (see Photograph X). It has been around almost as long as humans have been smoking cannabis and has a long history of medical use.

The ground bud can be smoked or vaporized. It is titrated at the same intervals as smoking bud and is also a much more concentrated form of cannabinoids and terpenes. The dose needs to be adjusted so as not to get too much medication with each inhalation as well. Cannabis bud and hashish are traditionally smoked or vaporized. There are no common high CBD*plus* varieties of hashish at this time.

Cannabis Oil

Cannabis oil is a highly concentrated form of cannabinoids in the oil base made by solvent extraction. They usually come in potency from 60-85 percent cannabinoids but have been reported to be as high as 99 percent cannabinoids (see Photograph XI). The oil can be consumed as an edible, but traditionally it is vaporized in a specially designed device that produces the very high temperatures necessary for vaporization of the extract for inhalation. This is a much higher temperature than is required to vaporize oil in diluents. Cannabis oils usually contain high amounts of THC and are used for recreational purposes. This formulation is very potent and complex to administer. There is also a huge potential for excessive euphoric and side effects from the THC and is therefore not recommended for medication administration.

The one exception is Rick Simpson Oil. Which is very high in THC and used for 60-90 days to treat late stage cancer.

https://www.leafly.com/news/cannabis-101/what-is-rick-simpson-oil

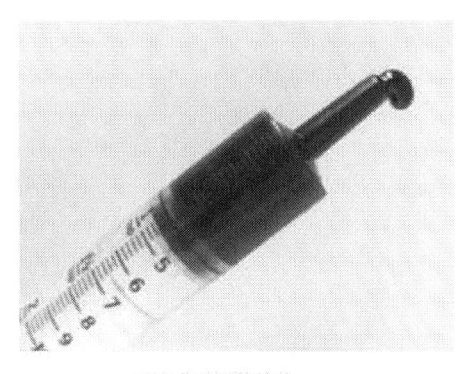

Photograph XI

Cannabis Tinctures and Extracts

Cannabis tinctures are made via alcohol extractions and are the vehicles for isolating oils such as coconut and vegetable oils. These liquids contain concentrated CBD*plus*, with or without THC, but also all of the other important organic chemicals in the plant, including other cannabinoids, terpenes and flavonoids. These liquids are often green from chlorophyll or honey colored and may have an unpleasant taste and smell. Some extraction techniques minimize the amounts of terpenes and chlorophylls in the tincture. Most tinctures and extracts are produced locally and do not meet the high level of consistency and quality control that come with large scale manufacturing organizations.

There are a handful of high quality, tested, certified, and contaminant-free CBD*plus* products available online or in stores around the country. Some of these brands include Absolute CBD™, Charlotte's Web™, and Hemp Meds™ (see Photograph XII). In addition, the website www.ProjectCBD.org and www.CBDoilreview.org provide up-to-date recommendations for high quality, available products.

Until cannabis was banned in 1937, pharmaceutical tinctures of cannabis oils were the second most common medication available at pharmacies. It is interesting to note in states where medical cannabis has been legal the longest, the trend been away from smoked or vaporized cannabis and toward an increasing cannabis being sold as a tincture or edible. This is because of the perceived negative effects from smoking and associated social issues with the aroma of the smoked or vaporized medicine.

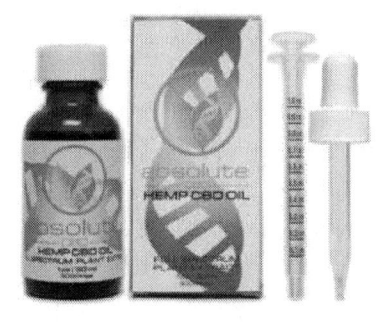

Photograph XII

www.TheHempDepot.com

Tinctures and extracts do not work as quickly as smoked or vaporized medicine but have a more rapid onset of action compared to other ingested forms of the medicine. The tincture is an approximately 75% alcohol vehicle that is delivered via a dropper under the tongue where more rapid absorption occurs via sublingual arteries. The drug misses much of the first-pass effect from the liver. Like smoked or vaporized medication, its effects come on quickly and dissipate rapidly in a few hours.

In addition, the precise measurements afforded by a dropper or oral syringe (see Photograph XII) and the precise concentrations of the tincture or extract lead to consistent dosing for the patient. It is important to advise the patient not to swallow the preparation, as this will cause it to go through the GI tract to the liver and undergo the 'first-pass effect'. If the tincture is added to a tea or liquid, then it absorbed as an "edible" form of the medication with the slow and gradual onset of effect associated with all cannabinoids that go through the GI system.

The type of cannabinoids present (THC, CBD and/or CBD*plus*) and their concentrations will be documented on packaging. Like strains of cannabis—unless high quality brands are purchased—these labels are often incorrect if the product does not have high standards of preparation, manufacturing and quality control.

Cannabis Butter and Edibles

Cannabis butter is a soft, light green, butter textured substance that is made from cooking the cannabis bud with butter to extract the cannabinoids into the butter. It is seldom eaten by itself but is used to cook and bake a wide variety of cannabis edibles. In addition, there are an increasing variety of candies and flavored drinks that have extracted cannabinoids in them.

The cannabinoids are digested in the gastrointestinal tract and go through the first pass effect of the liver. This means that the time it takes to have an effect is much longer (about one to two hours) and that the effects themselves last much longer (five to six hours). Furthermore, when THC is ingested and is metabolized by the liver it is actually converted to a different substance called 11-hydroxy-THC. This is many times more psychoactive than the delta-9-THC that is in inhaled cannabis. Although there is minimal research on the metabolism of CBD*plus,* it is suggestive that when ingested, most of the CBD*plus* will be broken down into inactive compounds by the first pass effect. Therefore, ingesting CBD*plus* is a much less effective way to receive the medication. Oromuscosal absorption (under the tongue) and inhalation (vaporizing) are the recommended ways to take CBD*plus* medications.

Edibles and cannabis butter have several positive aspects. They have a slow onset of action and prolonged duration or effect, which makes them good for chronic pain control or nighttime dosing. Edibles are hard to dose because of the large variation in the batches of cannabis butter that is produced in small operations. Also, the amount of active ingredients in the edible decreases with longer duration of exposure to stomach acids. The presence or absence of food in the stomach can likewise affect absorption and clinical effects.

Unlike CBD or CBDplus, eating too many milligrams of THC can cause dysphoria—a highly unpleasant sensation akin to agitation, panic, or impending doom. People will often go the emergency room when the dysphoria is very bad or prolonged. Be careful with edibles; especially when they are from small "mom and pop" manufacturers.

Like all products found in the dispensary, the amount of THC, CBD or CBD*plus* in the product may be incorrect due to problems with quality control and manufacturing in small start-up companies making these edibles. Once again, when dosing and titrating start with a low dose—or a small piece of the edible—

and increase slowly until you feel comfortable with the correct dose for the condition. Edibles can be hard to titrate because of the slow onset of action and long duration of effect. Oftentimes, there is markedly less cannabinoid in the product than the label says. There are few standards for labeling and packaging for these products. A recent informal analysis of several popular brands of edibles in Colorado found only a minute fraction of the cannabinoid in almost all of the products sold by several manufacturers.

In time, new regulations and enforcement will result in higher quality and standards for edibles. For the present time, however, the patient will have to become familiar with dosing different brands of edibles.

Patients like edibles; which, like tinctures, do not require any smoke or vapor and the associated tell-tale smell or respiratory tract irritation. They can be ingested anywhere and are reasonably priced compared to cannabis bud or hashish.

For example, of rapid onset of action, to reduce hunger pangs, inhalation of a vape is recommended, usually one to two inhalations. This usually will last up to 90 minutes.

For example, of long term action, a bedtime dose for continued control of blood sugar or blood lipids, use an extract under the tongue. This will usually last for 12-24 hours.

Packaging Issues

A safety issue has been recognized with edibles that contain THC. They usually come is simple packaging and they are usually tasty treats such as baked goods, candies or soft drinks. This has resulted in spike in the number of children mistakenly ingesting the edible and ending up in the emergency room. There are no reported deaths, but serious side effects from the euphoric effects have been reported. New laws are being enacted mandating packaging and requiring single wrap servings to prevent accidental excessive dosing. CBD*plus* only products, even in very high doses of hundreds of milligrams, have no appreciable side effects or euphoria.

Below (Photograph XIII) is an image of an example label for a cannabis medication. In this case, the label is for bud, and so it will show the amount of THC and CBD*plus* by percentage. It also shows that the product has passed a "Safety Screen" for microbes, fungi, and pesticides. If this label was on an extract or

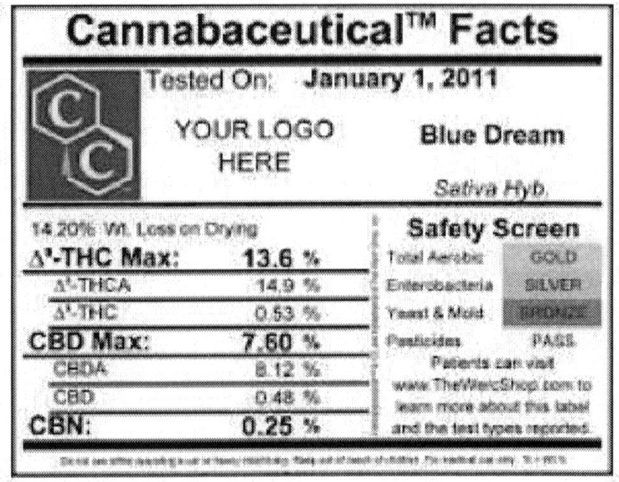

Photograph XIII

edible it wouldn't have a percentage of THC and CBD but would have the number of milligrams of CBD and THC per dose of serving. Labels in the near future are expected to also include the percentage or number of milligrams of THCV (CBD*plus*).

CBD*plus* Infused Topical Medications

Hemp oil that is high in CBD*plus* can be extracted and infused into a wide variety of vehicles, such as creams or lotions (water soluble), ointments or balms (fat soluble), sprays, lubricants, infused-rubbing alcohol or dermal patches that are applied to the skin.

Since cannabis oils are fat soluble, they don't penetrate very deeply into the tissues and tend to work just on the skin and in the tissue just under the skin. Due to the fact that there is little or no absorption of the cannabis into the bloodstream with topical preparations, there are none of the side-effects—such as euphoria, anxiety, or addiction—that people tend to worry about when using inhaled or ingested cannabis.

Cannabis-infused topicals have been used for hundreds of years and have been shown to be particularly useful for a wide array of skin conditions, fibrotic conditions just under the skin, and locally inflamed or arthritis joints.

There is no high-quality research on the topic of topical application of CBD*plus*. At this time, it is not clear what, if any, therapeutic benefits would be derived from using topical CBD*plus*. There is suggestive evidence in animal studies of CBD*plus* stimulating hair growth via blockade of CB1 receptors on hair follicles. CBD*plus* topicals are being looked for treatment of balding, alopecia areata and effluvium.

CBD*plus* Isolates Versus Whole Plant Extracts

The vast majority of CBD and CBD*plus* products available in stores or online are made with isolated CBD and CBD*plus*. This pure CBD*plus* has been extracted from the hemp oil and has only tiny amounts of the other cannabinoids and terpenes in the oil. The soon to be approved prescription medicine, Epidiolex(r), is 99% pure CBD oil. Usually, these isolates are very clear, as can be seen in photograph XIV. These pure isolates tend to have no smell or taste since CBD*plus* are odorless and tasteless.

The preferred CBD*plus* products, however, are not isolates, but are made from whole-plant extract. These extracts range from 3-20% CBD*plus* and the rest of the oil is non-THC cannabinoids, such as CBG, CBN, CBC and CBD and many terpenes. These whole-plant extracts tend to be dark green and has a fruity or earthy flavors and aromas from the terpenes (see Photograph XII).

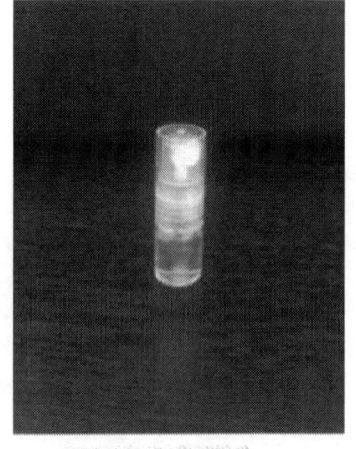

Photograph XIV

A 2015 study from Israel directly challenges one the main premises of the big pharmaceutical companies, that artisanal, botanical and whole-plant extracts are inherently inferior to pure isolates. The study was conducted by a one of the scientists who discovered the components of the ECS. The study showed that isolates of CBD*plus* have a "bell-shaped" curve when it comes to dosing. That is, as the dose of CBD*plus* gets bigger, there is more of a therapeutic benefit; however, at a certain dose the effects actually become less. Therefore, with isolates the goal is to find the "sweet spot" dose discussed in a later chapter. This need to find the "sweet spot" is not a good quality of a medicine, as there is only a narrow "window" for the correct dose, if the dose goes above that level, then the benefits rapidly decrease.

In the study they used a whole-plant extract that was 17.9% CBD with tiny percentages of many other cannabinoids and terpenes. This is similar to Charlotte's Web and Absolute CBD brand extracts. They compared this in mice to an isolate of CBD, which was similar to Epidiolex(r). The whole-plant extract had a direct dose dependent response to pain and inflammation. That is as the dose increased, so did the benefit. There was no drop off as the dose went higher. Of course, at a certain dose of CBD, there were no additional therapeutic benefits. This makes whole-plant extracts a preferable way to dose CBD*plus*. Researchers also found that a lower dose of CBD was needed to get the same benefits for pain or inflammation reduction, and they felt that the whole-plant extract was a superior medication due to the "Entourage Effect" of the other cannabinoids and terpenes on the ECS receptors.

CHAPTER 4: HOW SAFE IS CBD*PLUS*?

In this chapter, I will discuss how CBD*plus* has been shown to be very safe with none of the euphoria of getting 'high' or risk of dependency or addiction that is associated with THC.

Hemp Oil

CBD*plus* and CBD are legal and available in all 50 states without a prescription, as long as it comes from low-THC hemp plants that were grown under the auspices of the federal 2014 Farm Bill (and often a state hemp bill as well). When the oil is extracted from these low THC cannabis or hemp plants it is considered by the federal government as a nutritional supplement that is 'generally recognized as safe' (GRAS) by the FDA.

Extraction Techniques

There are several extraction techniques. Most of the time, for 99% pure CBD*plus* oil, the original hemp or cannabis oil has undergone four separate extraction techniques. The use of organic solvents, such as butane and propane, can leave behind a residue that is inhaled or ingested along with the CBD*plus*. It is recommended that only cold CO_2 extraction methods be used. But no matter what method is used, certified laboratory results of the cannabis bud, extract, or tincture should be available to the consumer either online or at the dispensary.

Contaminants

There are no federal and few and inconsistent state laws regarding testing for contamination of hemp or cannabis oil. In addition to the residues of organic solvents used to extract the oil from the plant material, there are several other significant contaminants to be concerned about. These include pesticides, heavy metals, microorganisms such as mold and aflatoxins from fungi. Repeated low level exposure to any of these contaminants can have serious health effects. Again, the dispensary should have laboratory results that certify the absence of heavy metals, pesticides, microorganisms, and fungi.

> CANNCON, Inc (www.jcanna.com) is a non-profit organization that was formed to provide high quality analytic testing to the medical cannabis community.
>
> The educational website www.MedicalJane.com has a detailed analysis, by state of the current situation with getting accurate laboratory testing of medical cannabis, or CBD*plus* extracts, and tinctures.

Consistency

Most bud that is high in a specific cannabinoid such as CBD*plus*, CBD, or THC will have significant variation in the potency from batch to batch. This is because cannabis is a plant and the amount of oil that it produces will naturally vary with different conditions. The edibles, tinctures and other products tend to be manufactured by small companies and can also have issues with significant variation in the product. For CBD*plus* or CBD only products this is not a huge concern, because if one batch is slightly weaker than another it will soon become apparent to the person using the medication and the dose can easily and safely adjusted. With THC, this is a different matter because significant changes in the THC can have result in major side effects and euphoria that do not occur with CBD*plus* only medication.

The few manufacturers of high quality CBD*plus* and CBD products test each batch for consistency and contaminants when the oil is initially processed and at the end of the manufacturing process. They also send batches of their products to independent laboratories for analysis.

A recent article in the Journal of the American Medical Association evaluated 84 CBD products from online stores, including extracts, vapes and edibles. They tested the products and compared what they found to what the label said. 43% of the products had less CBD than stated on the label, and only 31% had accurate labeling.

Side Effects

For the doses that are discussed in this book—5mg to 40mg a day—there are no real side effects. There are some pleasant effects associated, such as mood elevation, relief of anxiety, reduced inflammatory pain and stiffness from arthritis, and body relaxation. These pleasant side-effects are seen with CBD as well, but none of these side-effects impair the brain or one's ability to drive, think, operate devices, or are associated with cancer or other chronic disease.

There are reports that CBD*plus* will increase the intensity of the euphoria associated with THC. However, this occurs at higher doses of THCV (CBD*plus*) than are recommended in this book. Since these over-the-counter hemp oil products contain only minimal amounts of THC this is not an issue.

Allergy

Just like other weed pollen, such as ragweed, cannabis pollen may trigger an allergic reaction. There are hundreds of by-products in smoke that may trigger allergy. In addition, people may have an allergic reaction to contaminants such as mold, fungi and pesticides.

Although still uncommon, there are an increasing number of reports of allergy to cannabis bud and cannabis-based medications. The most common symptoms of allergy would be runny nose, nasal congestion, sneezing and a dry cough. Swelling and itching around the eyes and hives on the skin have also been reported. There have been very rare reports of severe anaphylactic allergic reaction after eating a cannabis edible.

Some studies have suggested that exposure to hemp pollen in large outdoor grows can result in people becoming allergic to cannabis pollen. If you think that you are having allergic reactions to cannabis bud or extract, you should discontinue using it and discuss it with your medical professional.

Special Groups of People

As we have discussed above, CBD*plus* is exceptionally safe, essentially has no side effects and can have significant health benefits for a wide variety of conditions. However, there are certain groups of people who should have focused discussion with their medical professional prior to considering taking CBD*plus*, CBD or cannabis products.

Pregnancy

Like most medications, there is very little research on the effects of CBD*plus*, CBD and THC during pregnancy. Approximately 2-5% of women report using cannabis during pregnancy. All of the cannabis oils are fat soluble and easily cross the placenta into the fetal blood supply. There are some animal studies that show that cannabis can affect fetal neurological development. One study in animals using very high doses of THC. that suggests that low birth weight and premature birth, and behavioral issues later in childhood. However, these were very high doses of THC.

This can be an issue since THC has been shown to be particularly useful for the treatment of 'morning sickness', which occurs in 70-80% of pregnancy women. This is especially true when other FDA approved medications don't work or can't be used during pregnancy. One study from 1994, was done of Jamaican mothers. The mothers used a home-remedy of cannabis to treat the morning sickness. They were compared to similar Jamaican mothers who didn't use any cannabis. The study found no differences in birth weight, premature delivery or behaviors in infancy and childhood.

Three large studies of British, Australian and Dutch women did not find any association with cannabis use during pregnancy and low birth weight or premature delivery.

There are two ongoing studies of child who were exposed to high doses of THC while their mothers were pregnant. There is a suggestion of increased behavioral issues, lower IQ and psychotic symptoms later in childhood. However, some of these effects may be due to the fact that the mothers also smoked and used alcohol during the pregnancy.

These studies are ongoing as more research on this topic clearly needs to be done. Like smoking cigarettes and drinking alcohol, the general advice is to refrain from using cannabis-based medication during pregnancy or while they are actively trying to get pregnant.

Breast Milk

All of the oils in cannabis are fat soluble and small quantities will therefore end up in a mother's milk. Like most medications, there is very little research on the effects of CBD*plus*, CBDV and THC on developing infants. However, one study did reveal that all of the oils and several of the metabolites in cannabis can end up in the breast milk.

One study even suggests that the daily use of THC by breastfeeding mothers could retard infant motor development. Another study found no effects on infants. These two studies both have problems and more high-quality research is needed in this area.

Studies are ongoing and more research on this topic needs to be done. Like smoking cigarettes and drinking alcohol, the general advice is to refrain from using hemp-based medication while breastfeeding.

Children

The brain continues to undergo important development up until age 25. The ECS in the brain is involved with laying down the correct nerve tracts in the brain. Excessive dosing of THC in animals has been shown to affect the normal development of several nerve systems in the brain. There is also evidence in humans that regular use of THC, especially in high levels, or the use of THC throughout the day, can cause structural changes in the brain which are associated with emotional and reasoning issues.

Unlike CBD*plus*, CBD has most of its effects outside of the brain, in the body's immune system. However, CBD does cross over into the brain and there are effects in the immune system cells in the brain from CBD. CBD has been used in high doses in high quality randomized clinical trials for the treatment of intractable seizures in infants and toddlers. These studies of these infants do not reveal any significant side effects from CBD. Even so, additional long-term studies are needed.

Elderly

The elderly population will probably benefit the most from CBD. CBD has many positive effects on conditions that are common in the elderly, such as arthritis, dementia, and cancer. Unlike THC, which can cause many unpleasant side effects, including anxiety, agitation, short-term memory loss, issues with balance and euphoria, CBD has minimal side effects and makes CBD an excellent adjunct medication for elderly patients.

Since very elderly patients metabolize medications differently than younger adults, it is recommended to start dosing at half the recommended dose and to move the dose up gradually in very old patients.

Other Medications

There are many medications that can interact with THC. Since THC has most of its effects in the brain, other medications that affect mood, balance, memory, or cause euphoria, can have synergistic effects when THC is also taken.

CBD*plus*, however, has almost no side effects and along with CBD and THC can inhibit the action of a very important enzyme system in the liver called P450. This enzyme system is involved with the metabolism and breakdown of 60% of the FDA approved medications that we use. There is a potential for slight increases in the blood levels of these medications with use of higher doses of CBD*plus*. For the vast majority of medications, this slight increase is not important. Although for some drugs, such as anticoagulant and anti-epilepsy drugs, this increase in blood level can have a serious effect.

Your medical professional can review which medications that you are taking and discuss using them in combination with CBD*plus*. Remember that vast majority of physicians and nurses have had no education about the ECS, THC, or CBD*plus*. So, you may want to have them follow the link below and read an excellent article on the subject of CBD*plus* and the P450 system at Project CBD.

> www.projectCBD.org/article/CBD-drug-interactions-role-cytochrome-p450

Alcohol

Alcohol consumption can cause euphoria, mood disturbances, balance and co-ordination—all of which can occur with THC. Alcohol used in high doses over a long period of time is associated with liver fibrosis and eventually potentially fatal cirrhosis. Once again, CBD does not have these side effects. In, fact CBD has been shown to decrease the brain degeneration associated with long-term alcoholism and reverse liver fibrosis in certain clinical situations. Studies in mice have shown that taking CBD oil after binge drinking had a protective effect on the liver. It has been recommended to take 20-40mg of CBD as a preventative; however, further studies need to be conducted.

Drug Addiction and Dependencies

Persons with a history of drug/alcohol addiction or dependency are strongly cautioned against using THC. This because up to 9% of persons using high doses of THC daily, on a long-term basis, may develop a dependency on THC. Being at an adolescent age or having a history of other addictions greatly increases the likelihood of developing THC dependency as well. Fortunately, THC dependency is much milder and easier to treat than other additions such as opioids or benzodiazepines. CBD*plus* and CBD do not cause a dependency or addiction, so this is not an issue when using CBD*plus*.

Schizophrenia or Psychosis

Using high doses of THC has been associated with temporary episodes of paranoia and psychotic behavior. There is some research that shows an association between recreational THC use and the onset of schizophrenia. Because of this information, persons with a family history of psychosis or a prior history of a psychotic episode should not use THC.

On the other hand, CBD has been shown to actually improve psychosis and is being evaluated for use as new type of anti-psychotic medication. Several promising studies in animals and humans have shown significant effects with schizophrenia and psychosis. It is not clear how CBD has these effects, but functional MRI studies of the brain have confirmed CBD has effects in the areas of the brain associated with psychosis. In addition, the temporary psychosis caused by excessive THC can be treated with a 100-22mg dose of pure CBD oil.

Side Effects Specific to CBD*plus*

Due to the heightened alarm over the use of Rimonabant, some have expressed concern that CBD*plus* may have some similar side-effects. Rimonabant is a synthetic cannabinoid and does not exist in nature. It was developed by the pharmaceutical industry in 2006 to help people lose weight. It is a negative or "inverse" blocker of the CB1 receptor; which means that it does exactly the opposite of what THC does. THC is a "positive" stimulator of the CB1 receptor. This drug was developed to increase metabolism and promote weight loss. However, after it was released in several European countries it was quickly revealed that it could cause significant depression and even suicide. It also caused nausea in a significant portion of users. Rimonabant was removed from the market in 2008. It was never approved for use by the FDA in the US.

CBD*plus* is a naturally occurring "neutral" blocker of the CB1 receptor. This means that it binds to the receptor and physically blocks ANA, 2-AG and THC from binding to the receptor. The net result is that it results increased metabolism, expenditure of energy, and homeostasis of blood sugar, and lipids. CBD*plus* does not have to side-effects of depression, suicidal thoughts or nausea that were strongly associated with the synthetic drug Rimonabant. Separately, CBD*plus* has been shown to work similarly to CBD and increase endocannabinoid tone at CB1 and CB2 receptors via inhibition of the breakdown of naturally occurring ANA and 2-AG.

CHAPTER 5: HOW TO USE CBD*PLUS*

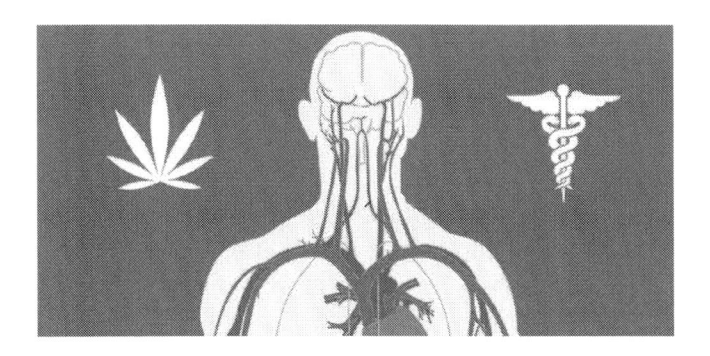

Start Low, Go Slow

CBD*plus* is very safe, non-addictive and does not cause euphoria. THC has issues with addiction and euphoria, as well as several other issues with anxiety, agitation, coordination and short-term memory. Due to the many potential problems of THC, any time medical cannabis is used that contains levels of THC of 3% or greater the medication needs to "start low" at a low dose and gradually "go slow", moving up the dose until the desired medical effect.

This is not the case with CBD*plus* only medications. In general, there will be a recommended dose range and you can start with this dose and increase as necessary based on the response. CBD*plus* is safe and without side-effects well into the 100mg range. However, for most conditions that I discuss in this book, the treatment will be less than 200mg a day.

Sweet Spot

When it comes to using THC, CBD, or CBD*plus* for medical purposes, a little is better than a lot. Most of the therapeutic effects from THC, CBD or CBD*plus* occur in ranges of a few milligrams. If you take too much, the excess amounts of THC, CBD, or CBD*plus* in the blood stream will literally flood the cannabinoid receptors (CB1 and CB2). These receptors are not flooded naturally; so when this occurs, the receptors tend to sink inside the cell and leave fewer receptors. This will result in more medication being necessary to get the same effect. When this occurs, it is called 'tolerance'.

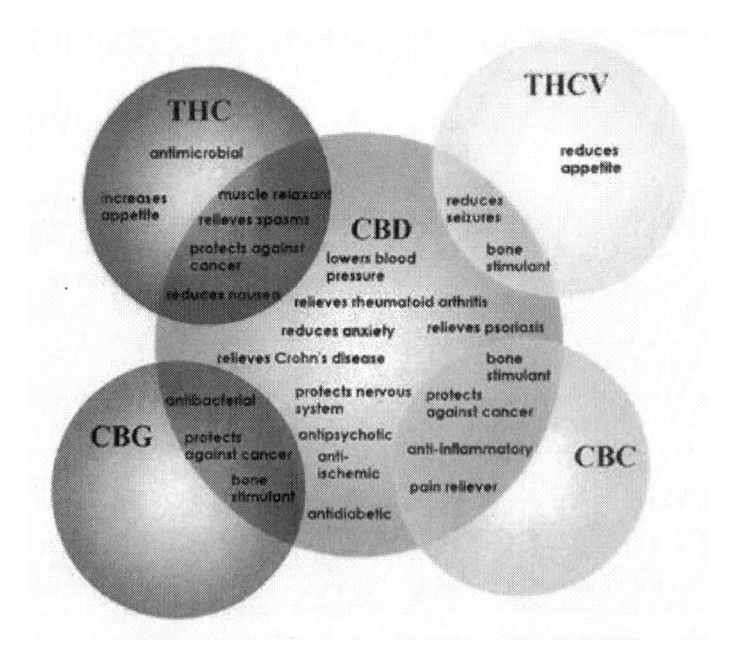

THC: antimicrobial, increases appetite, muscle relaxant, relieves spasms, protects against cancer, reduces nausea

THCV: reduces appetite, reduces seizures, bone stimulant

CBD: lowers blood pressure, relieves rheumatoid arthritis, reduces anxiety, relieves psoriasis, relieves Crohn's disease, bone stimulant, protects nervous system, protects against cancer, antipsychotic, anti-ischemic, anti-inflammatory, pain reliever, antidiabetic

CBG: antibacterial, protects against cancer, bone stimulant

CBC: (shown in diagram)

The goal when using CBD*plus* is to get to the "sweet spot". The "seet spot" is the blood level that is high enough to have a therapeutic effect but high enough to where it floods the receptors and leads to tolerance. The recommended doses of CBD*plus* in this book are designed to reach these "sweet spot" levels in an average adult. However, it is expected that most people will have to gradually titrate up to the "sweet spot" dose, from the initial or starting dose.

As the diagram above shows, each of the cannabinoids in hemp oil have their own specific therapeutic effects, but there is also some overlap with other cannabinoids.

Re-Evaluate

After starting CBD*plus* it is necessary to re-evaluate the condition to see if the dose of medication is having a desired and significant effect. Perhaps raising the dose a little will have more of a positive effect.

CBD and CBD*plus* are not like aspirin or blood pressure pills. Except for a few symptoms, you cannot expect a measurable effect until you have been taking the medication for several days. With CBD*plus* it really depends on which condition you are treating to determine how frequently you should increase the dose. Please see the dosing advice provided in each chapter on specific conditions such as weight loss, pre-diabetes, diabetes, blood lipids and fatty liver. Once you get to the dose that is working for you, then you can re-evaluate less frequently, such as every 3-6 months.

> A diary is a good way to track the progress of your dose or medication. Document the dose taken, the time of day and changes in symptoms experienced. After two weeks you can look at the diary to get an idea of how the dose is working and make

> adjustments accordingly. There are several free or inexpensive apps for smartphones that have diaries for medical cannabis, weight loss and symptoms.

Tips on Dosing CBD*plus*

Hemp oils, which includes CBD and CBD*plus*, are unlike almost all other medications. First, is it a plant extract that is often extracted and packaged without high levels of quality assurance. It can have contaminants such as leftover pesticides, extraction chemicals, heavy metals from the soil, and microbes such as fungi. There are dozens of CBD*plus* products on the market but only a small number that address all of these quality and consistency issues. I recommend The Hemp Depot, Green Roads, or Charlotte's Web Hemp products, because they have independent testing and certification of good manufacturing practices to insure safety and consistency. In addition, their products cost less or the same as inferior quality brands.

CBD*plus* is fat soluble, and therefore more difficult to absorb. Some brands are now making water-soluble CBD*plus* isolates but these don't have the terpenes and may not have the Entourage Effect. Once CBD*plus* is absorbed, most of it is metabolized before it ever gets a chance to have an effect. Because of this, the best type of CBD*plus* medication is a whole-plant extract, which insures that the oil is in a natural balance with the terpenes and other cannabinoids.

As discussed earlier, the CBD*plus* can be inhaled, usually through a vaporizer, for quick yet short term effects, to reduce hunger. For longer action—such as overnight—it can be absorbed by swishing on the inside of the mouth as discussed earlier.

Ingesting a CBD*plus* edible or swallowing the CBD*plus* extract is not recommended. After the CBD*plus* is ingested in goes into the intestinal tract and through the 'first pass effect' of the liver and most of the active medication is turned into inactive metabolites and excreted. This means only a small percentage, maybe 15%, of the medicine actually gets into the blood stream to do its work. Some available topical creams and patches purport to be effective in treating disease throughout the body and not just locally. However, because of the lack of high quality studies showing the absorption rates and efficacy at this time, none of these brands are recommended for effects, other than local application.

There are many ways to take your medicine, but the most recommended way is to vaporize CBD*plus* and inhale it for quick onset of action (10-20 minutes), and short duration of effect (90 minutes). Swish the CBD*plus* around under your tongue for slower onset (30-45 minutes) but longer-term effect (12-24 hours).

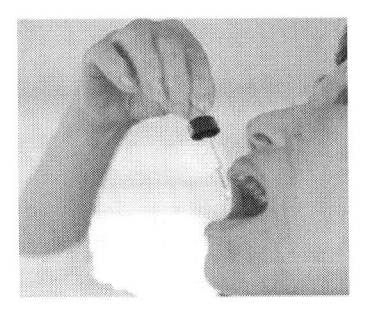

Before starting treatment with CBD*plus*, start using a "health diary". There are several apps for your smartphone available to track how your weight, appetite, blood sugars and blood fats respond to medication. Find the right one and start tracking your activity, dietary intake and hunger for a couple days before you start taking CBD*plus*. Based on what you read about the effects of *CBDplus* on hunger and dietary intake, try to identify a handful of specific goals that you would like to see from CBD*plus*, later on in the book. In addition to specific weight and diet goals, you may also want to track your general 'mood.'

For weight loss and appetite suppression, after four days of the same dose you can decide if you want to increase your dose in order to get more of an effect. You can keep increasing CBD*plus* dose every four days until you feel that you are at the maximum effect. Remember that because of the "sweet spot" on the dose curve, if you start taking too high of a dose it will result in you getting lesser medical effects.

With weight loss, you typically start at a specific dose—such as 5mg—at bedtime and increase it by 5mg every four days until you get to the "sweet spot" dose. Most of the people will respond to 20mg-40mg a day of CBD*plus*. The daily dose can be divided such as half an hour before each the two biggest meals of the day. Because blood lipids, blood sugar and fatty liver needs to be tested to determine one's clinical improvement, the doses are usually increased every 3 months or so after the doctor repeats the specific test and determines the effect of the CBD*plus*.

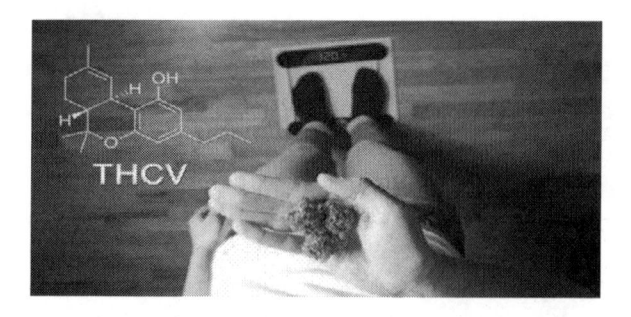

If you feel that you have received maximum benefit from the CBD*plus*, it is important to continue taking the dose on a long-term basis; although it is sometimes advisable to eventually taper off CBD*plus*. You may have reached a specific weight goal or control of blood sugar or lipids, so that the CBD*plus* dose can be tapered or stopped. If you are tapering of long term use of CBD*plus*, it would be advisable to cut the dose in half every four days until you get back to the starting dose, and then quit.

Where to Get CBD*plus* Medication

It is very important from whom you get your medication. Any medical cannabis products that contain THC will have to come from a state-approved dispensary. The staff at the dispensary are able to help you find the right type of medication, and method of taking the medication. In general, you will be able to buy one month of medical cannabis at a time. So, each month when you go back you can discuss how the medical cannabis that they have recommended is working for you.

> The following three websites list all of the state-approved dispensaries in your area.
>
> www.Leafly.com
>
> www.MarijuanaDoctors.com
>
> www.WeedMaps.com

CBD*plus* oil is often bought online, as it is legal in all 50 states and able to be shipped across state lines. Don't forget that the term 'CBD*plus*' is just used for this book; and when ordering CBD*plus* products in a store or online, you are looking for THCV, or tetrahydrocannabivarin. The important thing to remember is to select a high quality, contaminant-free product. There are dozens of websites selling CBD*plus* oil, but the vast majority of these are selling over-priced inferior products. Recently the FDA sent out 'cease and desist' warning letters to companies selling extracts of CBD and making health claims.

For several years I have been asked by patients and doctors to recommend one brand of CBD and CBD*plus* products. Because of the issues discussed above, I have been very hesitant to do this. However, I have evaluated three companies manufacturing processes, laboratory testing, good manufacturing practices certification and products and I now feel very comfortable recommending the following two THCV (CBD*plus*) manufacturers. Their products are available around the world in retail stores and through online purchases.

---

www.thehempdepot.org (Absolute Products)

www.CWhemp.com (Charlotte's Web Products)

The website www.CBDoilreview.org has some good information about many brands and CBD*plus* products. Also discounts on products are available through the website.

Drug Testing and CBD*plus* Use

A real and common concern among people using legal over-the-counter CBD and CBD*plus* products is whether it can cause a urine or hair drug test to become 'positive' for cannabis or THC. The answer is an emphatic 'no.' The tests that are conducted on hair and urine samples are very specific and test solely for THC and metabolites of THC. CBD*plus* and CBD are an entirely different chemicals and does not cross-react on the screening or confirmatory drug tests.

The real problem rests with attempts to buy a product that is supposed to have less than 0.3% THC in it to find out that it actually has a lot higher concentration of THC than expected. Using a product that is incorrectly labelled can and has resulted in a 'positive' drug test.

This is one more reason to only purchase CBD*plus* products that are from high quality manufacturers, such as The Hemp Depot, that have accurate labeling and testing of their products.

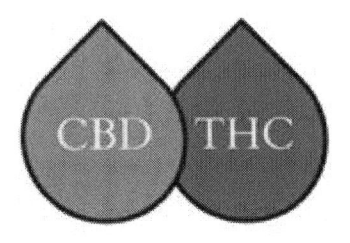

Getting Your Doctor Involved

Over 95% of doctors, pharmacists, and nurses never learned about the ECS in school and have little or no experience with hemp oil, CBD*plus*, CBD or medical cannabis. Instead of trying to educate your busy health care provider with a quick talk, I recommend you write down this website on a piece of paper and give it to the provider to look at when they have a moment. This is quick, concise, science-based discussion of the 'pros' and 'cons' surrounding medical cannabis and hemp oil. In my experience, almost every provider will want to start learning more about the ECS, THC, CBD, CBD*plus* after looking at this convincing site.

"The 10-Minute Summary," at ProCon.org.

(http://medicalcannabis.procon.org/view.resource.php?resourceID=142)

I have mentioned several times that your regular physician may have no knowledge or experience with using medical cannabis, CBD*plus* extract. If you can't convince your medical professional to help you add medical cannabis, CBD*plus* oil to your treatment, then you can find a compassionate, educated and experienced medical professional in your area at one of these three websites.

www.Leafly.com

www.MarijuanaDoctors.com

www.WeedMaps.com

The doctors that are listed at these websites have met certain criteria and are specialized in the use of THC, CBD, CBD*plus*. Make certain that they are willing to communicate with your regular medical provider, so that your care and medication use is coordinated correctly.

Section II:

Conditions treated with CBD*plus*

CHAPTER 6: DIABETES MELLITUS

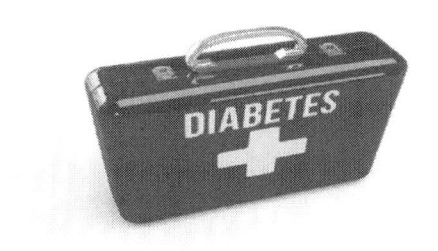

Personal Story

> A concerned wife of a man with diabetes came to see me. She and her husband were visiting from Georgia and wanted to get a medical cannabis card. She was going to use the card to get medical cannabis for her husband and bring it back to Georgia. I told her husband that he had a good chance of responding to a combination of CBD and CBD*plus*. I told him he didn't need a medical cannabis card. He could get all the high quality CBD*plus* and CBD oil she needed mailed right to their home in Atlanta. I gave him the name of a couple websites and I told the couple that CBD and CBD*plus* oils were available without a prescription and could be legally mailed right to their home.
>
> She felt a little silly for driving seven hours each way to find that out, so I didn't charge them for the consultation. I told him to make certain that his internist in Atlanta was involved with his care. I got a nice email from the wife a few months later and her husband was doing great.

Introduction

Diabetes mellitus refers to a group of metabolic disorders in which there are high blood sugar levels over a prolonged period of years. Symptoms of high blood sugar include unexplained rapid weight loss, frequent urination, increased thirst, and increased hunger. If left untreated, diabetes can cause many complications, some of them are life-threatening.

As of 2015, an estimated 415 million people had diabetes worldwide, with type 2 DM making up about 90% of the cases. This represents 8.3% of the adult population, with equal rates in both women and men. As of 2014, trends suggested the rate would continue to rise. Diabetes at least doubles a person's risk of early death. From 2012 to 2015, approximately 1.5 to 5.0 million deaths each year resulted from diabetes. The global economic cost of diabetes in 2014 was estimated to be U.S. $612 billion. In the United States, diabetes cost $245 billion in 2012.

Diabetes is due to either the pancreas not producing enough insulin or the cells of the body not responding properly to the insulin produced. There are three main types of diabetes mellitus:

- Type 1 DM results from the pancreas' failure to produce enough insulin. This form was previously referred to as "insulin-dependent diabetes mellitus" (IDDM) or "juvenile diabetes". The cause is unknown and it usually starts in childhood.

- Type 2 DM begins with insulin resistance, which is a condition where cells fail to respond to insulin properly. As the disease progresses, a lack of insulin may also develop. This form was previously referred to as "non-insulin-dependent diabetes mellitus" (NIDDM) or "adult-onset diabetes". The most common cause is excessive body weight and insufficient exercise.

- **Gestational diabetes** is the third main form and occurs when pregnant women without a previous history of diabetes develop high **blood sugar** levels.

Acute complications can include **diabetic ketoacidosis,** hyperosmolar hyperglycemic state, or death. Serious long-term complications include **cardiovascular disease,** stroke, chronic kidney disease, foot ulcers, and damage to the eyes.

Prevention and treatment involve maintaining a healthy diet, regular physical exercise, a normal body weight, and avoiding use of tobacco. Control of blood pressure and maintaining proper foot care are important for people with the disease. Type 1 DM must be managed with insulin injections. Type 2 DM may be treated with medications with or without insulin. Insulin and some oral medications can cause low blood sugar. **Weight** loss **surgery** in those with **obesity** is sometimes an effective measure in those with type 2 DM. Gestational diabetes usually resolves after the birth of the baby.

Pre-diabetes

Pre-diabetes, which is very common and may affect as many as 86 million Americans, is when your blood sugar is higher than it should be, but not high enough to be considered diabetes mellitus. Normal fasting blood sugar levels should be 100 or less, and diabetes is diagnosed when the blood sugar is consistently above 126. So, pre-diabetes is diagnosed when a blood sugar level is between 101-125. It is a wake-up call to lose weight, exercise and modify unhealthy eating habits. Pre-diabetes will usually progress to full blown Type 2 diabetes if not addressed.

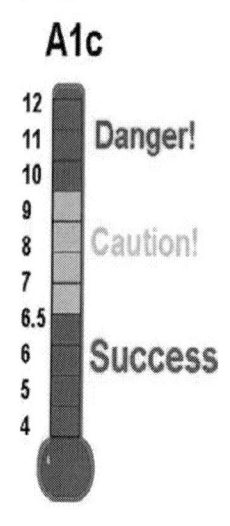

A1c

12
11 **Danger!**
10
9
8 Caution!
7
6.5
6 **Success**
5
4

To determine if blood sugar levels are consistently running high the medical provider will order a Hemoglobin A1C test, abbreviated HgbA1C. In a person with normal blood sugars it will be 5.6% or less, and in diabetes it is 6.5% or higher. So, pre-diabetes is confirmed if the HgbA1C test is from 5.7% to 6.4%.

Taking twice daily CBD*plus* may help the cells in the pancreas naturally improve blood sugar control in persons with pre-diabetes.

Your medical provider can perform lab tests to determine the presence of pre-diabetes and diabetes. These tests are done fasting.

SIGNS of Diabetes Mellitus:

unexplained rapid weight loss

frequent urination

increased thirst

increased hunger

CBD*plus* Studies

Studies in mice of CBD*plus* showed that increasing doses improved fasting plasma glucose and glucose tolerance following an oral glucose challenge test. This was especially true when the CBD*plus* was administered twice daily. Furthermore, the studies in mice showed that CBD*plus* increased energy expenditure, particularly in very obese mice with a genetic tendency towards obesity. Also, CBD*plus* was effective at reducing liver triglyceride levels related to high blood fats.

In genetically normal mice with diet-induced obesity, CBD*plus* improved glucose tolerance and increased insulin sensitivity and reduced insulin-resistance. The conclusion of the mice studies was that CBD*plus* is a new potential treatment against obesity-associated glucose intolerance and was pharmacology different from that of the drug Rimonabant, discussed in the previous chapter.

GW Pharmaceuticals is a UK-based drug company that specializes in the development of drugs based on cannabis oils. GW has recently commenced a 12-week randomized, double blind, placebo-controlled study of THCV (CBD*plus*) to treat Type 2 diabetes. The primary objective of this study is to compare the change in blood sugar control in participants with Type 2 diabetes when treated with one of three doses of CBD*plus* or placebo as add-on therapy to the diabetes drug metformin. The safety and tolerability of CBD*plus* compared with placebo will also be assessed.

This study follows positive findings reported in November 2012 from a Phase 2a exploratory study, showing evidence of anti-diabetic effects of CBD*plus* and supporting advancement of CBD*plus* into further clinical development. The 2012 Phase 2a trial had a total of 62 Type 2 diabetes patients and showed that CBD*plus* produced a variety of desirable anti-diabetic effects including reduced fasting plasma glucose levels, an increase in fasting insulin, improved pancreatic beta-cell function, increased serum adiponectin, reduced systolic blood pressure, and reduced serum IL-6 levels. Several of these findings are consistent with pre-clinical data suggesting that CBD*plus* protects the insulin-producing cells of the pancreas and is a highly desirable feature for a new anti-diabetic medicine. Not to mention, CBD*plus* also increases insulin sensitivity and reduces fasting plasma glucose levels.

Dosing

CBD*plus* is used to help blood sugar control in Type 2 diabetes and especially in pre-diabetes. It is only for use in adults and should always be used under the supervision of an experienced medical provider.

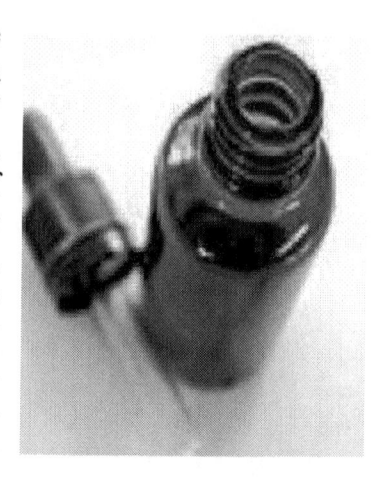

Based on the clinical research data gleaned from the GW pharmaceutical trials, the starting dose of CBD*plus* is 2mg under the tongue, twice daily, 12 hours apart. The dose can be gradually increased based on blood sugar levels and other tests of blood sugar control. The maximum expected dose is 16mg twice daily.

Generally, the 2mg twice daily dose is taken for 3 months and the medical provider will re-measure the fasting blood sugar and HgbA1C levels. The studies show that there is a dose-related response; therefore, increasing the dose of CBD*plus* is expected to have superior results. The dose can be increased to 4mg twice daily after 3 months and doubled again to 8mg and then to a maximum of 16mg twice daily if the medical provider agrees.

Treatment Doesn't Always Work

Medicine is an art more than it is a science. Sometimes the recommended treatment doesn't work. It may not work because the dose wasn't correct. Or, it may not work because the underlying condition causing the symptoms is more severe than originally thought.

Start out with the recommended CBD*plus* extract dose. If the maximum doses of CBD*plus* extract isn't providing enough relief of cravings, it is time to go back to your physician for some advice.

Involving Medical Professionals

Diabetes Mellitus is a significant and potentially life-threatening condition. There are many serious complications that can occur in the eyes, kidneys, and extremities. Due to the complexity and severity of diabetes, patients with the disease should always work closely with their medical provider to determine if adding CBD*plus* or medical cannabis is appropriate. The medical providers usually have little or no training on the subject and often won't actually recommend the CBD*plus*. However, then may give their permission to add CBD*plus* to the patient's treatment.

> If your regular doctor won't work with you to dose medical cannabis you can find a compassionate, experienced licensed clinician who will, in your area at the following websites:
>
> www.Leafly.com
>
> www.MarijuanaDoctors.com
>
> www.WeedMaps.com

CHAPTER 7: HIGH CHOLESTEROL AND BLOOD LIPIDS

Introduction

Hyperlipidemia is abnormally elevated levels of any or all lipids in the blood. This includes elevated cholesterol and/or triglycerides.

Nearly 37% of Americans have cholesterol or triglyceride levels where medical providers would recommend drug treatment. A little more than half of those who need cholesterol medication are taking it.

Hyperlipidemias are divided into primary and secondary subtypes. Primary hyperlipidemia is usually due to familial or genetic causes, while secondary hyperlipidemia arises due to other underlying causes such as diabetes. Lipid and lipoprotein abnormalities are common in the general population and are regarded as modifiable risk factors for heart disease and heart attack due to their influence on atherosclerosis or hardening of the arteries.

In addition, some forms hyperlipidemia may predispose to acute pancreatitis. Your medical provider can perform lab tests to determine the presence of hyperlipidemia. These tests are done fasting.

In general, there are two broad types of cholesterol that can be measured:

LDL or the "bad" cholesterol is the fraction of the total cholesterol that forms the plaque that can clog the arteries. Optimal LDL level is less than 130mg per dL, or less than 100 per dL in persons with other risks for heart disease.

> HDL or the "good" cholesterol keeps cholesterol from building up in our arteries. Optimal HDL level is greater than 40 mg per dL in men and greater than 50 mg per dL in women.

Diet and exercise can improve mild cases of hyperlipidemia but usually the medical provider will need to use medication to lower unhealthy levels.

SIGNS of Hyperlipidemia:

Rarely yellowish fatty growths around the eyes or joints

Generally, people have no symptoms and require a fasting blood test

---

CBD*plus* Studies

Activation of the cannabinoid receptor CB1 has been shown to induce fatty liver disease and hyperlipidemia. Studies in genetically obese mice have shown that high doses of CBD*plus* improve liver triglyceride levels and reduce evidence of hepatic damage

Studies of mice with diet-induced obesity showed that CBD*plus* used in a high dose, once a day, improved hyperlipidemia by decreasing total cholesterol, and causing a healthy increase in the HDL/LDL ratio. Interestingly enough, these effects were seen with the once a day, and not with the twice daily administration protocol.

Studies in humans include a randomized, double-blinded, and placebo-controlled trial of sixty-two adults. The subjects were given one of the following dosages twice daily for the duration of 13 weeks: 100mg of CBD; 5mg of THCV (CBD*plus*); 5mg of CBD plus 5mg of THCV (CBD*plus*); 100mg of CBD plus 5mg of THCV (CBD*plus*); or a placebo.

The results showed that CBD*plus* treatment led to an increase in protein Apo A (a major constituent of the 'good cholesterol' HDL) concentrations compared to baseline and placebo. CBD*plus* was also associated with a reduction in plasma glucose concentration, which was in line with significant increases in other measures of blood glucose control. The researchers were concerned that the dose of CBD*plus* was not enough to get maximum clinical effects. The results suggest that CBD*plus* is well-tolerated and could have significant therapeutic effects in the control of blood glucose of patients with type 2 diabetes. Larger clinical trials are now warranted to fully assess its therapeutic and adverse effects over a longer period of time.

Dosing

Starting adult dose (not recommended in children) 5mg of CBD*plus* extract under the tongue twice daily. After three months the medical provider will re-assess fasting blood lipids to determine if the dose needs to be increased. May increase to 10mg, then 15mg and finally 20mg dose twice daily depending on response measured on the blood tests. Once maximum benefit has been achieved with a certain dose, maintain that dose. Maximum dose 20mg twice daily.

Treatment Doesn't Always Work

Like I always say, medicine is an art more than it is a science. Sometimes the recommended treatment doesn't work. It may not work because the dose wasn't correct, or because the underlying condition causing the symptoms is more severe than originally thought.

Start out with the recommended CBD*plus* extract dose. If the maximum doses of CBD*plus* extract isn't providing enough relief of cravings, it is time to go back to your medical provider for some advice.

Involving Medical Professionals

Elevated cholesterol and lipids can be serious or may represent a more serious underlying condition. Starting CBD*plus* for treatment of elevated cholesterol or lipids should be considered only after discussion with your cardiologist or primary care physician. As is unfortunately usually the case, most physicians will have very little knowledge of CBD*plus* or medical cannabis, and their use with cholesterol and lipids. However, it is important to give your doctor the opportunity to assist you controlling your blood fats. Do not attempt to suddenly decrease or discontinue your prescriptions medications. Involve your doctor while you gradually titrate the dose of CBDplus to control your blood fats.

> If your regular doctor won't work with you to dose medical cannabis you can find a compassionate, experienced licensed clinician who will, in your area at the following websites:
>
> www.Leafly.com
>
> www.MarijuanaDoctors.com
>
> www.WeedMaps.com

CHAPTER 8: WEIGHT LOSS

Introduction

Being overweight or fat is having more body fat than is optimally healthy and is especially common where food supplies are plentiful and lifestyles are sedentary.

As of 2003, excess weight reached epidemic proportions globally, with more than 1 billion adults being either overweight or obese. In 2013, this increased to more than 2 billion individuals and have been observed across all age groups.

A healthy body requires a minimum amount of fat for proper functioning of the hormonal, reproductive and immune systems, as thermal insulation, as shock absorption for sensitive areas and as energy for future use. Although, the accumulation of too much storage fat can impair movement, flexibility, and alter the appearance of the body.

Body Mass Index (BMI)

Body Mass Index (BMI) is a measurement of a person's weight with respect to his or her height. It is more of an indicator than a direct measurement of a person's total body fat. BMI, more often than not, correlates with total body fat. This means that as the BMI score increases, so does a person's total body fat. The WHO defines an adult who has a BMI between 25 and 29.9 as overweight - an adult who has a BMI of 30 or higher is considered obese - a BMI below 18.5 is considered underweight, and between 18.5 to 24.9 a healthy weight. BMI is used by healthcare professionals to screen for overweight and obese individuals. The BMI is used to assess a person's health risks associated with obesity and overweight.

For example, those with a high BMI are at risk of:

- high blood cholesterol or blood fats
- type 2 diabetes
- heart disease
- stroke
- high blood pressure
- certain cancers
- gallbladder disease
- sleep apnea and snoring
- premature death
- osteoarthritis and joint disease

BMI Calculator

Body Mass Index (BMI) Chart for Adults

■ Obese (>30) ■ Overweight (25-30) ■ Normal (18.5-25) ■ Underweight (<18.5)

HEIGHT in feet/inches and centimeters

WEIGHT lbs (kg)	4'8" 142cm	4'9" 147	4'10" 150	4'11" 152	5'0" 155	5'1" 157	5'2" 160	5'3" 163	5'4" 165	5'5" 168	5'6" 170	5'7" 173	5'8" 175	5'9" 178	5'10" 180	5'11" 183	6'0" 185	6'1" 188	6'2" 191	6'3" 193	6'4" 196	6'5"
260 (117.9)	58	56	54	53	51	49	48	46	45	43	42	41	40	38	37	36	35	34	33	32	32	31
255 (115.7)	57	55	53	51	50	48	47	45	44	42	41	40	39	38	37	36	35	34	33	32	31	30
250 (113.4)	56	54	52	50	49	47	46	44	43	42	40	39	38	37	36	35	34	33	32	31	30	30
245 (111.1)	55	53	51	49	48	46	45	43	42	41	40	38	37	36	35	34	33	32	31	31	30	29
240 (108.9)	54	52	50	48	47	45	44	43	41	40	39	38	36	35	34	33	33	32	31	30	29	28
235 (106.6)	53	51	49	47	46	44	43	42	40	39	38	37	36	35	34	33	32	31	30	29	29	28
230 (104.3)	52	50	48	46	45	43	42	41	39	38	37	36	35	34	33	32	31	30	30	29	28	27
225 (102.1)	50	49	47	45	44	43	41	40	39	37	36	35	34	33	32	31	31	30	29	28	27	27
220 (99.8)	49	48	46	44	43	42	40	39	38	37	36	34	33	32	32	31	30	29	28	27	27	26
215 (97.5)	48	47	45	43	42	41	39	38	37	36	35	34	33	32	31	30	29	28	28	27	26	25
210 (95.3)	47	45	44	42	41	40	38	37	36	35	34	33	32	31	30	29	28	28	27	26	26	25
205 (93.0)	46	44	43	41	40	39	37	36	35	34	33	32	31	30	29	29	28	27	26	26	25	24
200 (90.7)	45	43	42	40	39	38	37	35	34	33	32	31	30	30	29	28	27	26	26	25	24	24
195 (88.5)	44	42	41	39	38	37	36	35	33	32	31	31	30	29	28	27	26	26	25	24	24	23
190 (86.2)	43	41	40	38	37	36	35	34	33	32	31	30	29	28	27	26	26	25	24	24	23	23
185 (83.9)	41	40	39	37	36	35	34	33	32	31	30	29	28	27	27	26	25	24	24	23	23	22
180 (81.6)	40	39	38	36	35	34	33	32	31	30	29	28	27	27	26	25	24	24	23	22	22	21
175 (79.4)	39	38	37	35	34	33	32	31	30	29	28	27	27	26	25	24	24	23	22	22	21	21
170 (77.1)	38	37	36	34	33	32	31	30	29	28	27	27	26	25	24	24	23	22	22	21	21	20
165 (74.8)	37	36	34	33	32	31	30	29	28	27	27	26	25	24	24	23	22	22	21	21	20	20
160 (72.6)	36	35	33	32	31	30	29	28	27	27	26	25	24	24	23	22	22	21	21	20	19	19
155 (70.3)	35	34	32	31	30	29	28	27	27	26	25	24	24	23	22	22	21	20	20	19	19	18
150 (68.0)	34	32	31	30	29	28	27	27	26	25	24	23	23	22	22	21	20	20	19	19	18	18
145 (65.8)	33	31	30	29	28	27	27	26	25	24	23	23	22	21	21	20	20	19	19	18	18	17
140 (63.5)	31	30	29	28	27	26	26	25	24	23	23	22	21	21	20	20	19	18	18	17	17	17
135 (61.2)	30	29	28	27	26	26	25	24	23	22	22	21	21	20	19	19	18	18	17	17	16	16
130 (59.0)	29	28	27	26	25	25	24	23	22	22	21	20	20	19	19	18	18	17	17	16	16	15
125 (56.7)	28	27	26	25	24	24	23	22	21	21	20	20	19	18	18	17	17	16	16	16	15	15
120 (54.4)	27	26	25	24	23	23	22	21	21	20	19	19	18	18	17	17	16	16	15	15	15	14
115 (52.2)	26	25	24	23	22	22	21	20	20	19	19	18	17	17	16	16	16	15	15	14	14	14
110 (49.9)	25	24	23	22	21	21	20	19	19	18	18	17	17	16	16	15	15	15	14	14	13	13
105 (47.6)	24	23	22	21	21	20	19	19	18	17	17	16	16	16	15	15	14	14	13	13	13	12
100 (45.4)	22	22	21	20	20	19	18	18	17	17	16	15	15	14	14	14	13	13	12	12	12	12
95 (43.1)	21	21	20	19	19	18	17	17	16	16	15	15	14	14	13	13	13	12	12	12	12	11
90 (40.8)	20	19	19	18	18	17	16	16	15	15	15	14	14	13	13	13	12	12	12	11	11	11
85 (38.6)	19	18	18	17	17	16	16	15	15	14	14	13	13	13	12	12	12	11	11	11	10	10
80 (36.3)	18	17	17	16	16	15	15	14	14	13	13	13	12	12	11	11	11	11	10	10	10	9

Note: BMI values rounded to the nearest whole number. BMI categories based on CDC (Centers for Disease Control and Prevention) criteria.

www.vertex42.com   BMI = Weight[kg] / (Height[m] x Height[m]) = 703 x Weight[lb] / (Height[in] x Height[in])   © 2009 Vertex42 LLC

Rimonabant: A Problematic Cannabinoid Weight Loss Drug

Rimonabant (Acomplia®, Zimulti®, Rimoslim®) was a weight loss drug that was first approved in Europe in 2006. It caused weight loss in a novel way using the endocannabinoid system (ECS). Instead of stimulating CB1 receptors in the brain like THC, it did exactly the reverse and decreased ECS activity. This resulted in several effects related to increased energy metabolism and decreased appetite. The net result was on average about two to two and a half pounds of weight loss per month. Although it was good a causing weight loss, it unfortunately had serious and sometimes life-threatening psychiatric side-effects, including suicide, and was therefore withdrawn worldwide in 2008.

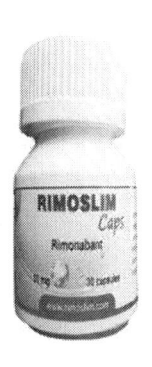

Rimonabant was never approved in the United States, even though it was submitted to the Food and Drug Administration (FDA) for approval in the United States in 2005. In 2007, the FDA's Endocrine and Metabolic Drugs Advisory Committee (EMDAC) concluded that Sanofi-Aventis failed to demonstrate the safety of Rimonabant and voted against recommending the anti-obesity treatment for approval and two weeks later the company withdrew the application.

In October 2008, the European Medicines Agency recommended the suspension of Acomplia® after the Committee for Medicinal Products for Human Use (CHMP) had determined that the risks of Rimonabant outweighed its benefits due to the risk of serious psychiatric problems, including suicide. In November 2008, an advisory committee in Brazil recommended suspension as well. The same month, Sanofi-Aventis suspended sale of the drug worldwide and the EMA approval was withdrawn in January 2009. The same year, India also prohibited the manufacture and sale of the drug. When the EMA reviewed post-marketing surveillance data, it found that the risk of psychiatric disorders in people taking Rimonabant was doubled.

Data from clinical trials submitted to regulatory authorities showed that Rimonabant caused depressive disorders or mood alterations in up to 10% of subjects and suicidal ideation in around 1%.

Additionally, nausea and upper respiratory tract infections were very common adverse effects, occurring in more than 10% of people. Other adverse effects, occurring in between 1% and 10% of people, include gastroenteritis, anxiety, irritability, insomnia and other sleep disorders, hot flushes, diarrhea, vomiting, dry or itchy skin, tendonitis, muscle cramps and spasms, fatigue, flu-like symptoms, and increased risk of falling.

Rimonabant Studies

Rimonabant is an inverse stimulator of the CB1 receptor and many of the good therapeutic effects of CBD*plus* are similar to Rimonabant. However, the nausea, seizure and psychiatric side-effects have not been seen with use of CBD*plus*, most likely because it is neutrally blocking the CB1 receptor and doesn't actively stimulate effects of the receptor. Most of the synthetic drugs, such as Rimonabant, are developed by pharmaceutical companies to look and act like the natural cannabinoids in hemp oil. However, when the pharmaceutical companies invent a new cannabinoid structure they are able to patent it and make significant profit being the only company allowed to sell the drug. Unfortunately, this profit-minded approach to medication has resulted in more than a few very bad outcomes.

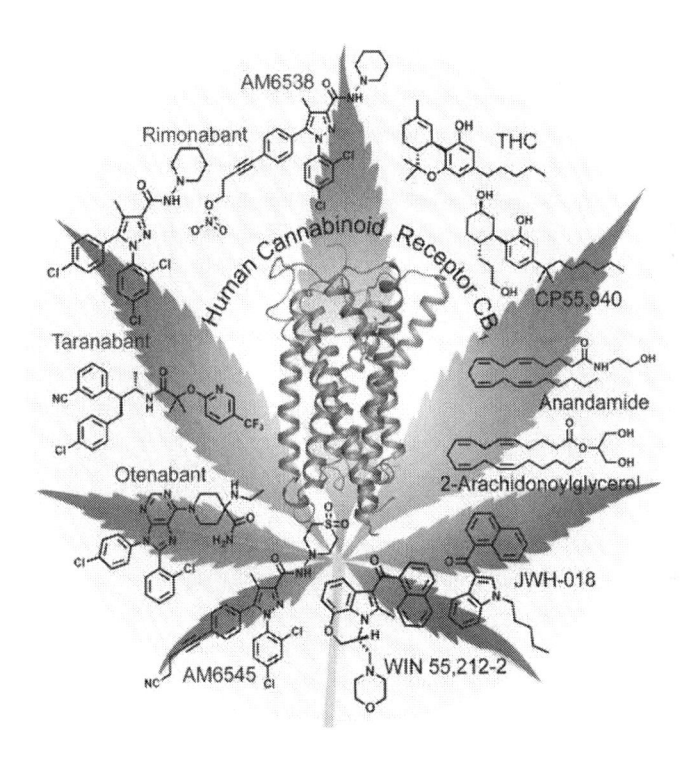

Rimonabant studied its efficacy in reducing obesity in diet-induced obese mice. This mouse model is widely used for research on the human obesity syndrome. During a 5-week treatment, Rimonabant showed reduction in food intake and marked but sustained reduction of body weight (-20%) and adiposity (-50%) over 5 weeks that increased as the dose of Rimonabant increased. Furthermore, Rimonabant corrected the blood sugars caused by insulin resistance and lowered plasma leptin, insulin, and free fatty acid levels. The studies confirmed that all of the effects of Rimonabant was via the CB1 receptors of the ECS.

Subsequent work showed that the anti-obesity effect of Rimonabant was also associated with improved blood lipids in a manner seemingly independent of the weight loss actions of the drug. Rimonabant treatment significantly reduced the high-fat diet-induced elevations in leptin, insulin and glucose. Although it did not modify HDL cholesterol, it had modest effects on total cholesterol and significantly reduced triglycerides and LDL cholesterol, thus increasing the HDL/LDL ratio.

Rimonabant is scientifically known as an "inverse" or negative CB1 stimulator. It does the inverse, or opposite, of what endocannabinoids like ANA, 2-AG and THC do. Thus, it has the opposite effects of ANA, 2-AG and THC; all of which are positive CB1 stimulators. As will be discussed in more detail later on, CBD*plus* is a "neutral" CB1 blocker; meaning, it attaches to the CB1 receptor like a lock in a key hole, but it neither locks or unlocks it. It simply blocks other stimulators of CB1, like ANA, 2-AG and THC, from fitting into the "key hole." If the receptor is blocked from ANA, 2-AG or THC then appetite stimulating effects of substances are blocked as well.

The net effect has been that CBD*plus* can increase energy expenditure and reduce appetite in the same way Rimonabant did, even though it doesn't cause the psychiatric, seizure threshold and nausea side-effects that are associated with inverse or negative stimulation of the CB1 receptor.

Rimonabant was extensively investigated in four randomized, double-blinded, placebo-controlled phase 3 clinical trials recruiting more than 6,000 overweight or obese patients whose weight at the start of the studies was on average 207lbs to 229lbs. Each of the four studies on Rimonabant showed significant reductions in body weight and waist circumference over a 1 to 2-year period.

Rimonabant also improved cardiometabolic risk factors, including triglycerides, blood pressure, insulin resistance, C-reactive protein levels, and HDL cholesterol concentrations in both non-diabetic and type 2 diabetic overweight/obese patients. Weight loss of 5-10% of body weight after one year of Rimonabant treatment was significantly greater in patients treated with Rimonabant. Rimonabant 20mg per day produced significantly greater improvements than placebo in waist circumference, HDL-cholesterol, triglycerides, and elevated blood sugar due to insulin resistance, and prevalence of the metabolic syndrome. The effects of Rimonabant 5mg per day were of less clinical significance.

Although Rimonabant was generally well-tolerated, later reports showed the use of Rimonabant was associated with psychiatric side effects including anxiety, depression, and suicidal thoughts. The adverse psychiatric events were observed in 26% of the participants in the Rimonabant group compared with 14% in the placebo groups and the risk of depressive symptoms was estimated at 2.5-fold higher in treated patients.

Other Drugs Like Rimonabant

Taranabant is a second drug that is an "inverse" CB1 blocker that has also been assessed in large scale clinical trials over a one-year period and showed nine pounds of weight reduction compared to placebo, similar to Rimonabant. However, psychiatric side effects were observed in all studies with Taranabant using both high and low doses. For this reason, psychiatric side effects are considered a class issue for first generation "inverse" CB1 blockers. As a consequence, the development of other similar drugs has been halted by pharmaceutical companies.

Other Drugs Like THCV (CBD*plus*)

A synthetic drug developed known as PIMSR is much like THCV (CBD*plus*), as well as a neutral CB1 blocker. It is basically the drug Rimonabant that has been modified to look more like THCV (CBD*plus*). In 2012, a study was done using PIMSR in mice on a high fat diet for 14 weeks. The mice were given a high dose of PIMSR for 28 days. They showed a 27% weight loss (vs 7% for control mice) and a persistently lower food intake. The adiposity index dropped to 40% of the treated mice. These mice also showed improved glycemic control in measures of glucose resistance, insulin sensitivity, blood sugar levels and elevated levels of insulin. Furthermore, there was improved blood lipid profiles with reduced serum triglycerides and cholesterol levels while HDL/LDL ratio improved.

PIMSR is closely related to CBD*plus* and has none of the depression or psychiatric issues that are associated with the inverse CB1 blocker Rimonabant.

The Anti-Munchies from CBD*plus*

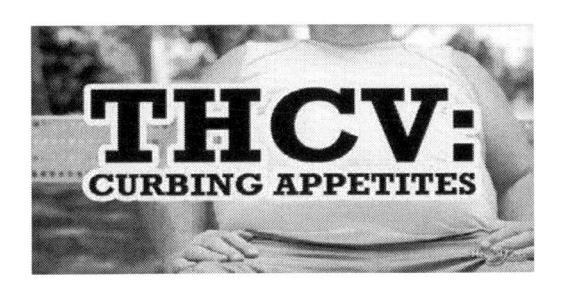

THCV: CURBING APPETITES

Most people are familiar with the munchies that is associated with using cannabis. This is the greatly increased appetite and actual craving for food that often accompanies using THC and is why medical cannabis is so useful with cancer patients. Not only does it take chemotherapy-induced nausea and vomiting away, but it actually stimulates cravings to eat.

Aroma and Taste

The munchies represent several phenomena going on in the brain and the body. THC stimulates the nerves in our olfactory bulb. This a small pea-like structure at the root of our nose, near our brain. THC increase our ability to smell food and improves the actual taste of the food. CBD*plus* sits on the CB1 receptors in the brain and physically blocks THC and our naturally occurring ANA and 2-AG from being able to stimulate these parts of our brain. The net result of using CBD*plus* is decreased olfactory stimulation from food aromas.

Visual Appeal

When we see delicious food a center in our brain called the nucleus accumbens is stimulated and releases dopamine. This causes the sensation of pleasure that comes when we eat especially tasty food. When we have THC in our body there is a greater release of the pleasurable dopamine from the nucleus accumbens when we eat. So, when someone is using THC the pleasure they associate with seeing, smelling, and tasting food is greatly enhanced. When CBD*plus* is occupying the CB1 receptors of the nucleus accumbens, there is significantly less release of dopamine in response to pleasurable appearance, aromas or taste of food.

Stomach Grumbling

Finally, we have many CB1 receptors on our hypothalamus. When we have THC in our body, the hypothalamus messages result in increased amounts of the hormone ghrelin being released in our stomach. Ghrelin stimulates hunger sensation and is a hormone that is produced in the stomach—especially when the stomach is empty. After the stomach is full (stretched), the production of ghrelin stops. Ghrelin is released into the blood stream and sends messages to the hypothalamus to increase the sensation of hunger and increases gastric acid secretion and gastric motility (stomach rumbling) to prepare the stomach for food intake as well.

Ghrelin actually makes our stomach rumble or growl. It is often this physical sensation of our stomach growling that makes people break their diet and start eating. Beyond the role in meal initiation, ghrelin is also involved in long-term body-weight regulation. Ghrelin levels circulate in relation to fat (energy) stores. Our ghrelin levels changes in response to body-weight alterations. Ghrelin crosses the blood-brain barrier and stimulates food intake by acting on several classical body-weight regulatory centers, including the hypothalamus, hindbrain, and mesolimbic reward system. Chronic ghrelin administration increases body weight via diverse, concerted actions on food intake, energy expenditure, and fuel utilization. Administration of drugs that block the effects of ghrelin reduces food intake and body weight. *CBDplus* reduces ghrelin release and therefore, decreases hunger pangs and stomach rumbling.

Feeling Full

Another hormone that is involved with appetite and fat storage is leptin. This hormone is produced by fat cells and is involved with telling the brain that we are satiated or full. There is some evidence to show that leptin also works via the ECS. Leptin reduces the desire for food intake and increases energy used by the body. Like ghrelin, leptin works via the hypothalamus and is reduced in response to CBD*plus*.

Decreasing Fat Storage

Fat cells, called adipocytes, are used to store extra energy for later use. Our blood sugar is converted into fatty acids which are stored in adipocytes. These fat cells respond to a locally produced hormone known as adiponectin that regulates the storage of extra energy into fat. The adipocytes have CB1 receptors on them and stimulation of these receptors results in decreases release of adiponectin. This decreases the storage of blood sugar into fat. CBD*plus*, which blocks CB1 receptors, increases release of adiponectin, which decreases the amount of blood sugar made by the liver, and suppresses storage of blood sugars into fat.

Animal Studies of THCV (CBD*plus*)

As I have mentioned earlier, CBD*plus* (THCV) is a neutral antagonist, or blocker of the CB1 receptors. It in animal studies it has been shown to produce decreased appetite and eating and body weight reduction in lean mice. Results from other animal experiments have shown that THCV (CBD*plus*) can suppress food consumption and body weight in non-fasted mice. However, like Rimonabant, THCV (CBD*plus*) did not reduce food intake and body weight in obese mice, even though it did improve elevated blood sugar in these animals. Furthermore, THCV (CBD*plus*) did not reduce food deprivation-induced food intake in mice.

Animal studies only provide suggestive evidence of the therapeutic benefit of a drug. In this case these animal studies suggest that the CBD*plus* may be most beneficial in persons trying to prevent the onset of obesity or help in mild obesity. The studies also show that CBD*plus* will not reduce the appetite in people who have been food deprived or starved.

The endocannabinoid system has been identified as playing a significant role in the control of appetite as well as glucose metabolism, and

Rimonabant was the first in a new class of agents that appears to work by selectively blocking the cannabinoid-1 receptors in the endocannabinoid system.

> CBD*plus* causes weight loss by blocking the CB1 receptors of the ECS in the brain to:
>
> Make food look, smell and taste less appealing
>
> Decrease stomach rumbling and hunger pangs
>
> Makes person feel full, and satiated
>
> Increase energy expenditure of the body

Other Nutraceuticals That Help with Weight Loss, Blood Sugar and Lipids

CBDV

There's good news for those looking to lose weight. Cannabidivarin, abbreviated CBDV, is another minor cannabinoid in hemp oil which has shown to work similarly to CBD*plus*. It is a natural appetite suppressant with none of the side effects that are inherent in most pharmaceutical treatments.

Curcumin

Several spices have been shown to exhibit activity against obesity through antioxidant and anti-inflammatory mechanisms. Among them, curcumin, a yellow pigment derived from the spice turmeric (an essential component of curry powder), has been investigated most extensively as a treatment for obesity and obesity-related metabolic diseases. Curcumin directly interacts with adipocytes, pancreatic cells, hepatic stellate cells, macrophages, and muscle cells. These curcumin-induced alterations reverse insulin resistance, hyperglycemia, hyperlipidemia, and other symptoms linked to obesity. Other structurally similar nutraceuticals derived from red chili, cinnamon, cloves, black pepper, and ginger, also exhibit effects against obesity and insulin resistance.

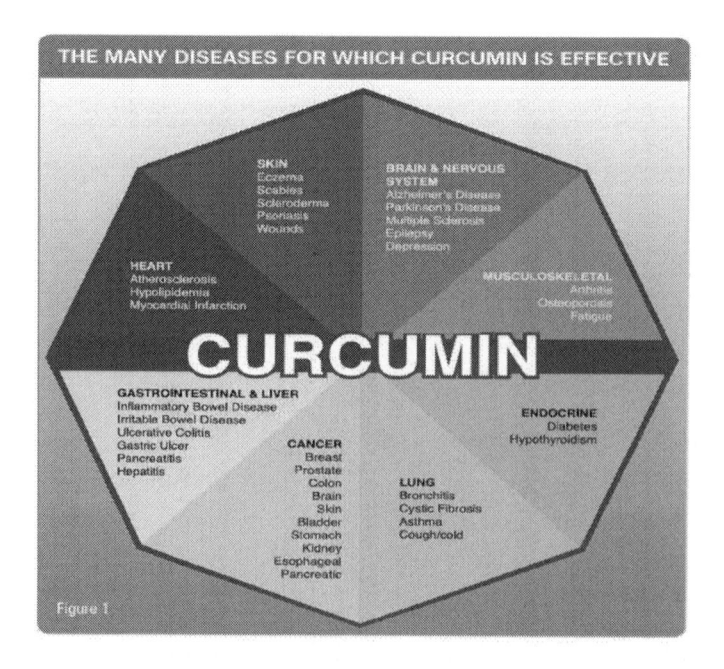

THE MANY DISEASES FOR WHICH CURCUMIN IS EFFECTIVE

CURCUMIN

SKIN
Eczema
Scabies
Scleroderma
Psoriasis
Wounds

BRAIN & NERVOUS SYSTEM
Alzheimer's Disease
Parkinson's Disease
Multiple Sclerosis
Epilepsy
Depression

HEART
Atherosclerosis
Hypolipidemia
Myocardial Infarction

MUSCULOSKELETAL
Arthritis
Osteoporosis
Fatigue

GASTROINTESTINAL & LIVER
Inflammatory Bowel Disease
Irritable Bowel Disease
Ulcerative Colitis
Gastric Ulcer
Pancreatitis
Hepatitis

CANCER
Breast
Prostate
Colon
Brain
Skin
Bladder
Stomach
Kidney
Esophageal
Pancreatic

ENDOCRINE
Diabetes
Hypothyroidism

LUNG
Bronchitis
Cystic Fibrosis
Asthma
Cough/cold

Figure 1

<u>Always Involve Your Medical Provider</u>:

If you're already taking a medication to help control your blood sugar levels, you shouldn't use curcumin supplements without talking with your doctor.

Combining these treatments may cause your blood sugar to drop, causing dizziness, blurred vision, fatigue, hunger, shaking or excessive sweating. Your doctor may need to reduce the amount of diabetes medication you are taking to counteract the effects of curcumin. People who are sensitive to curcumin may develop a skin rash or breathing problems after taking it. Otherwise, curcumin is usually well tolerated when used appropriately.

Recommended Daily Dose:

Curcumin is fat soluble and does not dissolve well in water-based solutions. It is also poorly absorbed after ingestion. Therefore, enhanced curcumin is recommended. This means that the curcumin has been modified so that it is more water-soluble, or nano-particalized to improve absorption in the GI tract. There are also combined products with piperine, or phosphatidylcholine. The recommended daily dose of curcumin that is enhanced for GI tract absorption is 500mg a day.

Cinnamon

A recent study found that when rats paired high-fat foods with cinnamon, they weighed less and had less belly fat than the rodents that didn't take cinnamon supplements. Other studies suggest cinnamaldehyde, the essential oil that gives cinnamon its flavor, helps mice eat less and ward off weight gain. Although, researchers weren't sure if it would hold true for humans.

Recently, researchers at the University of Michigan Life Sciences Institute treated human fat cell samples with cinnamaldehyde, and the study in the journal *Metabolism* has some promising findings. This new research discovered that cells treated with cinnamaldehyde started expressing more metabolism-boosting genes and enzymes. The cinnamon compound prompted fat cells to keep on burning instead of going into storage, so the researchers think it could help fight against obesity. Like CBD*plus*, cinnamaldehyde (the active ingredient in cinnamon) works by increasing metabolism.

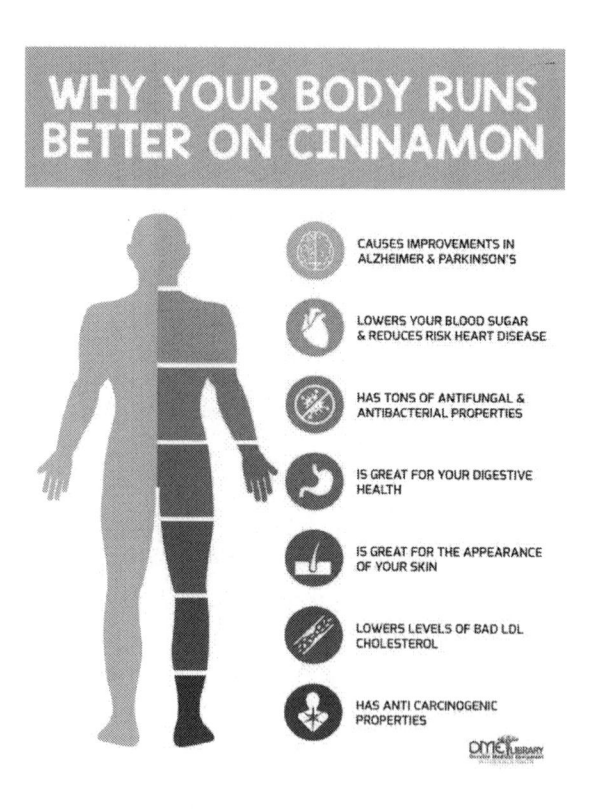

WHY YOUR BODY RUNS BETTER ON CINNAMON

- CAUSES IMPROVEMENTS IN ALZHEIMER & PARKINSON'S
- LOWERS YOUR BLOOD SUGAR & REDUCES RISK HEART DISEASE
- HAS TONS OF ANTIFUNGAL & ANTIBACTERIAL PROPERTIES
- IS GREAT FOR YOUR DIGESTIVE HEALTH
- IS GREAT FOR THE APPEARANCE OF YOUR SKIN
- LOWERS LEVELS OF BAD LDL CHOLESTEROL
- HAS ANTI CARCINOGENIC PROPERTIES

The active ingredients in cinnamon inhibit numerous digestive enzymes, such as alpha-glucosidase, sucrase and potentially pancreatic amylase causing a decrease of the glucose from the carbohydrates in the meal going into the body.

Another compound in cinnamon methylhydroxychalcone polymer, abbreviated MHCP, acts as like insulin on fat cells by aiding in the insulin resistance seen in pre-diabetes, diabetes and the metabolic syndrome. When ingested in human trials, cinnamon shows much promise in reducing blood glucose levels and sometimes markers of lipid metabolism (LDL, triglycerides, and total cholesterol). There are also intervention studies noting improved insulin sensitivity with cinnamon extract, possibly vicariously through the reduced blood glucose levels.

There are two types of cinnamon: ceylon and cassia cinnamons. They both look and taste the same. However, Ceylon cinnamon is always a better supplemental option than cassia cinnamon, due to the lower coumarin content. Using cassia cinnamon as a daily supplement in strongly advised against because of the potential toxic effects of coumarin in cassia cinnamon.

Always Involve Your Medical Provider:

If you're already taking a medication to help control your blood sugar levels, you shouldn't use cinnamon supplements without talking with your doctor. Combining these treatments may cause your blood sugar to drop severely, causing dizziness, blurred vision, fatigue, hunger, shaking or excessive sweating. Your doctor may need to reduce the amount of diabetes medication you are taking to counteract the effects of cinnamon. People who are sensitive to cinnamon may develop a skin rash or breathing problems after taking cinnamon. Otherwise, cinnamon is usually well tolerated when used appropriately.

Recommended Daily Dose:

The standard dose for anti-diabetic purposes is 1,000-6000mg of cinnamon daily to be taken with carbohydrate containing meals. There are a variety of products available that provide Ceylon cinnamon is pre-packaged doses to take with meals that contain carbohydrates.

Green Tea Catechins and Caffeine

Green tea (*Camellia Sinensis*) catechins mixed with caffeine have been proposed as nutraceutical for prevention and treatment of obesity. When not present with caffeine, it is known as Green Tea Extract (GTE). These catechins-caffeine mixtures, work better for weight loss than GTEs alone. The two together seem to counteract the decrease in metabolic rate that occurs during weight loss.

Their effects are of particular importance during weight maintenance after weight loss. Limitations for the effects of green tea catechins are moderating factors such as genetic predisposition related to a gene known as COMT, habitual caffeine intake, and ingestion combined with dietary protein. In conclusion, a mixture of green tea catechins and caffeine has a beneficial effect on body-weight management, especially by sustained energy expenditure and fat oxidation.

Always Involve Your Medical Provider:

If you're already taking a medication to lose weight you shouldn't use these supplements without talking with your doctor. People who are sensitive to catechins or caffeine may develop a skin rash or breathing problems after taking it. Otherwise, this supplement is usually well tolerated when used appropriately.

Recommended Daily Dose:

Supplements are compared to standard catechin known as EGCG. 400-500mg EGCG equivalent a day are recommended.

Gut Microbiota and Pre-biotics

Gut flora, gut microbiota or gastrointestinal microbiota is the complex community of microorganisms that live in our digestive tracts, mostly in the colon. In humans, the gut microbiota has the largest numbers of bacteria and the greatest number of species compared to other areas of the body. In humans the gut flora is established at one to two years after birth, and by that time the intestinal epithelium and the intestinal mucosal barrier that it secretes have co-developed in a way that is tolerant to, and even supportive of, the gut flora and that also provides a barrier to pathogenic organisms.

There is a mutually beneficial relationship between some gut flora and the human body. Intestinal bacteria also play a role in synthesizing vitamin B and vitamin K as well as metabolizing several nutrients. In fact, dysregulation of the gut flora has been correlated with a host of inflammatory and autoimmune conditions.

The composition of human gut microbiota changes over time, when the diet changes, and as overall health changes. A systematic review from 2016 examined the preclinical and small human trials that have been conducted with certain commercially available strains of probiotic bacteria and identified those that had the most potential to be useful for certain central nervous system disorders.

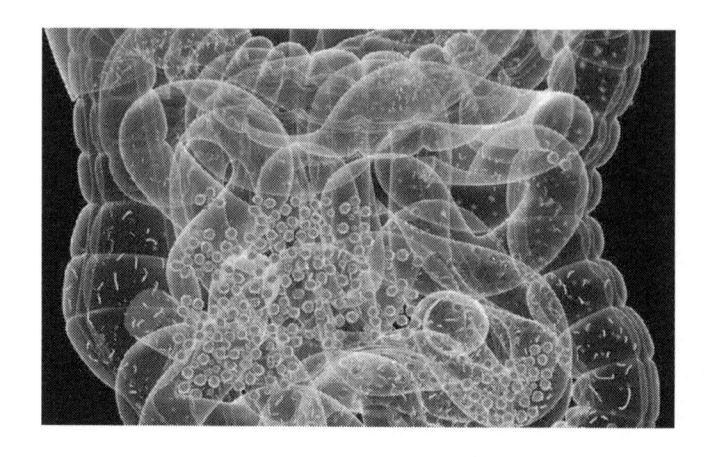

The bacteria that inhabit the intestines, are central to the pathogenesis of obesity. A review of 43 studies showed that calorie restrictive diets decreased the microbiota abundance, correlated with nutrient deficiency rather than weight loss. The impact of bariatric surgery on the gut flora depended on the given technique and showed a similar effect to calorie restricted diets. Probiotics differed in strain and duration with diverse effects on the microbiota and they tended to reduce body fat. Prebiotics were shown to contribute to the gut barrier and improving metabolic outcomes. All of the interventions under consideration had impacts on the gut microbiota, although they did not always correlate with weight loss. These results show that restrictive diets and bariatric surgery reduce microbial abundance and promote changes in microbial composition that could have long-term detrimental effects on the colon. In contrast, prebiotics might restore a healthy microbiome and reduce body fat.

Pre-biotics, such as Inulin (not insulin) various oligosaccharides are readily available. In addition to helping with obesity, they have been shown to have anti-inflammatory effects for inflammatory bowel diseases such as Crohn's and colitis.

<u>Recommended Daily Dose</u>:

There is no broad scientific consensus on a recommended daily serving amounts of the various pre-biotics. This is expected to change within the next five years as research and studies continue. The US Government's Dietary Guidelines for 2015-2020 recommend a range of 25-40 grams per day. The typical American diet probably is providing about 15 grams a day. So, one heaping tablespoon of a pre-biotic supplement, about 15 grams, is a good start. If there are no untoward symptoms after a week at this dose, the dose can be doubled to 15 grams twice a day, or even 30 grams, two heaping tablespoons once a day.

Chromium

Most often manufactured as chromium picolinate, chromium is a trace element that may be deficient in persons with diabetes. It has been suggested that chromium supplements may increase insulin sensitivity and improve glucose tolerance in patients with type 2 diabetes. Chromium's main mechanism is directly tied to chromodulin. Chromodulin, a protein, has to do with stimulating insulin production. If this protein is impaired, insulin's ability to work in the body is greatly reduced. A meta-analysis of randomized controlled trials investigating the effects of chromium supplementation on glucose and insulin response in healthy individuals and those with diabetes showed a modest but significant improvement in glycemic control in the latter, but not in the former. The American Diabetes Association's official position is that there is inconclusive evidence for the benefit of chromium supplementation in diabetes.

Always Involve Your Medical Provider:

If you're already taking a medication to help control your blood sugar levels, you shouldn't use curcumin supplements without talking with your doctor. Combining these treatments may cause your blood sugar to drop, causing dizziness, blurred vision, fatigue, hunger, shaking or excessive sweating. Your doctor may need to reduce the amount of diabetes medication you are taking to counteract the effects of curcumin. People who are sensitive to curcumin may develop a skin rash or breathing problems after taking it. Otherwise, chromium picolinate is usually well tolerated when used appropriately.

Recommended Daily Dose:

Chromium supplementation typically consists of 1,000 mcg of chromium picolinate, taken in at least two doses throughout the day.

Fiber

Fiber is a natural agent which slow carbohydrate absorption. Most notably are glucomannan and chlorogenic acid, both which are likely responsible for the reduction in diabetes risk associated with heavy coffee intake; and legume-derived α-amylase inhibitors.

A recent review of 44 studies found that while 39% of fiber treatments increased satiety, only 22% actually reduced food intake. If we break it down further, it seems that the more viscous a fiber is, the better it is at reducing appetite and food intake.

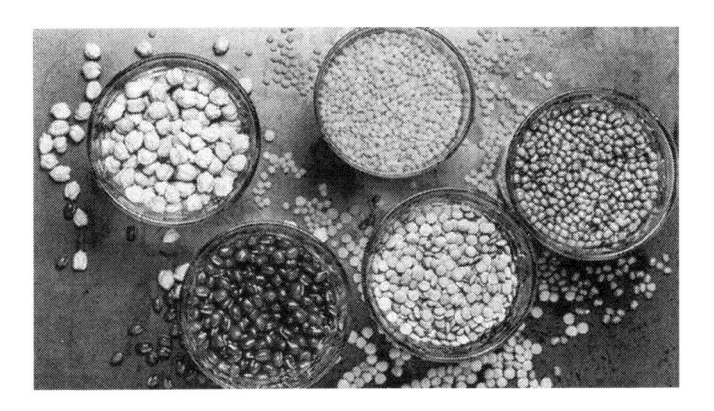

Put simply, the viscosity of a substance refers to its resistance to stress - as in, the "thickness" of a liquid. For example, honey is much more viscous than water. Viscous soluble fibers such as pectins, β-glucans, psyllium, glucomannan and guar gum all thicken in water, forming a gel-like substance that "sits" in the gut. This gel slows down the emptying of the stomach and increases the time it takes to digest and absorb nutrients. The end result is a prolonged feeling of fullness and a significantly reduced appetite.

There is some evidence that the weight loss effects of fiber target the belly fat specifically, which is the harmful fat in the abdominal cavity that is strongly associated with metabolic disease. Several forms of dietary fiber have been used as complementary or alternative agents in the management of the metabolic syndrome. Epidemiologic studies suggest an inverse relation of dietary fiber intake and body weight. However, randomized controlled studies suggest only minor effects on weight loss for commonly used dietary fiber supplements.

Recommended Daily Dose:

There is a wide variety of fiber supplements available. The dose to treat chronic constipation is much higher that the doses used for preventive purposes. When using fiber as a dietary supplement. In general, the dose is one tablespoonful in 8oz of water one two several times a day. It is recommended that the directions that come with the products are followed.

Treatment Doesn't Always Work

Medicine is an art more than it is a science. Sometimes the recommended treatment doesn't work. It may not work because the combination of medications wasn't correct, or it may not work because the underlying condition causing the weight gain is more severe than originally thought.

Involving Medical Professionals

It is important to give your doctor the opportunity to assist you controlling your weight. This is especially true, if several months and different efforts have been unsuccessful. Do not attempt to suddenly decrease or discontinue your prescriptions medications. Involve your doctor and ask her to help you gently taper off the prescription medications, why you gradually titrate the dose of CBD*plus* and the other wonderful nutraceuticals.

CHAPTER 9: FATTY LIVER DISEASE

Introduction

Fatty liver is a reversible condition wherein pockets of triglyceride fat accumulate in liver cells. Despite having multiple causes, fatty liver can be considered a single disease that occurs worldwide in those with excessive alcohol intake and the obese (with or without effects of insulin resistance). The condition is also associated with other diseases that influence fat metabolism. When this process of fat metabolism is disrupted, the fat can accumulate in the liver in excessive amounts, resulting in a fatty liver. It is difficult to distinguish alcoholic fatty liver disease, which is part of alcoholic liver disease, from nonalcoholic fatty liver disease (NAFLD), considering that both look the same of diagnostic studies and under a microscope.

The accumulation of fat in alcoholic or non-alcoholic fatty liver disease may also be accompanied by a progressive inflammation of the liver (hepatitis). This more severe condition may be termed either alcoholic steatohepatitis or non-alcoholic steatohepatitis.

The presence of non-alcoholic fatty liver disease (NAFLD in obesity has been linked to the worsening of the metabolic syndrome, including the development of insulin resistance and cardiovascular disease. Currently, there are few options to treat NAFLD, including life style changes and insulin sensitizers, such as CBD*plus* and other nutraceuticals discussed in the weight loss chapter.

Fatty liver

Synonyms Fatty liver disease (FLD), hepatic steatosis, simple steatosis

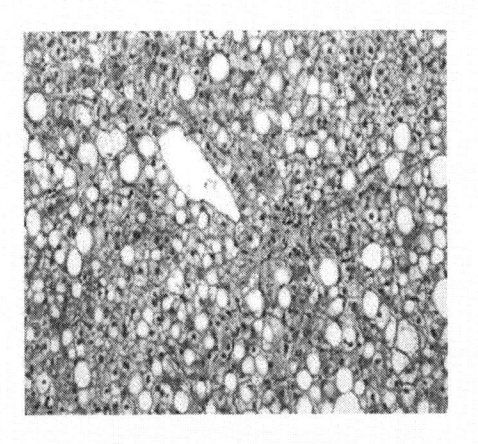

Micrograph showing a fatty liver (macrovesicular steatosis), as seen in non-alcoholic fatty liver disease. Trichrome stain.

PIMSR, discussed in an earlier chapter, is very similar to THCV (CBD*plus*). It was studied in very high doses in mice and shown dramatic positive effects in reducing weight, food intake, and aid in weight loss as well as in improve blood sugar control and blood lipid control in high fat diet-induced obese mice. The mice study also showed increased liver enzymes in the blood and evidence of liver injury with chronic administration.

The researchers felt that this was due to the very high levels of the PIMSR that were administered. It is unlikely that liver irritation will occur with CBD*plus*. In fact, in a separate study of PIMSR 3-day administration of PIMSR in C57BL/6J mice, hepatic steatosis from an acute administration of high of ethanol was significantly reduced. Also, it partially prevented alcohol-induced increases in ALT, AST, and

LDH. The differences in ALT levels with obese and non-obese mice under different test paradigms are unlikely to be due to neutral antagonism itself since other neutral antagonists (AM6545) do not exhibit liver injury.

Cannabinoids are a group of compounds acting primarily via CB1 and CB2 receptors. The expression of cannabinoid receptors in normal liver is low or absent. However, many reports have proven up-regulation of the expression of CB1 and CB2 receptors in hepatic myofibroblasts and vascular endothelial cells, as well as increased concentration of endocannabinoids in liver in the course of chronic progressive liver diseases. It has been shown that CB1 receptor signaling exerts profibrogenic and proinflammatory effects in liver tissue, primarily due to the stimulation of hepatic stellate cells, whereas the activation of CB2 receptors inhibits or even reverses liver fibrogenesis.

Doses of CBD*plus* for Fatty Liver Disease

CBD*plus* Extract

Starting adult dose (not recommended in children) 10mg of CBD*plus* extract under the tongue (oromuscosal absorption), morning, afternoon and bedtime. Do not increase dose until your medical provider has assessed the effects of several months use at this dose.

Liver and Milk Thistle

Milk thistle has been used for a number of purposes including treatment of liver disease, prevention and treatment of cancer, and supportive treatment of poisoning from death cap mushrooms; however, clinical study results were described as heterogeneous and contradictory. A 2007 Cochrane Review included eighteen randomized clinical trials which assessed milk thistle in 1088 patients with alcoholic and/or hepatitis B or C virus liver diseases. It questioned the beneficial effects and highlighted the lack of high-quality evidence. The review concluded that more good-quality, randomized clinical trials are needed. Cancer Research UK say that milk thistle is promoted on the internet for its claimed ability to slow certain kinds of cancer, but that there is no good evidence in support of these claims. Milk thistle may appear to stimulate prolactin due to possibly estrogenic activity.

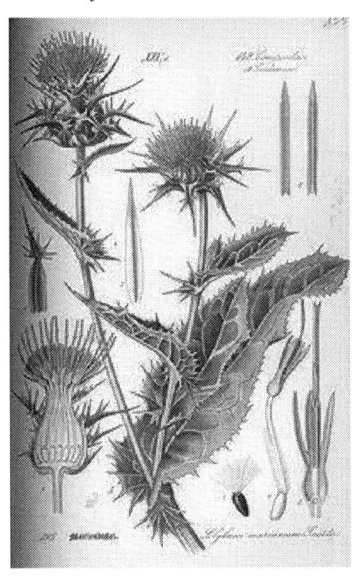

In 2015, a team of Egyptian scientists shed new light on silymarin's mechanism of action in a study on liver fibrosis in rats. The scientists concluded that silymarin conveys anti-fibrogenic effects by modulating cannabinoid receptor activity in the liver. Both types of cannabinoid receptors, CB1 and CB2, are expressed in the liver where they mediate opposing functions. Activating CB1 has a pro-fibrogenic effect, while activating CB2 has the opposite effect and reduces fibrosis. Silymarin blocks CB1 while turning on CB2 and is a perfect combination for treating hepatic fibrosis and chronic liver disease. The Egyptian study concludes that silymarin "strongly upregulates CB2 expression and downregulates CB1 expression. These effects may be partially responsible for the strong hepatoprotective effect of silymarin."

Tetrahydrocannabivarin (THCV) is an intriguing compound unique to the cannabis plant which interacts with the cannabinoid receptors in a similar way by blocking CB1 stimulation while boosting CB2 receptor stimulation. THCV-rich cannabis would likely benefit people with liver disease by working through some of the same molecular channels as Milk Thistle. Meanwhile, pharmaceutical researchers are seeking to develop synthetic, receptor-selective drugs that differentially engage both CB1 and CB2, much like THCV and silymarin.

Treatment Doesn't Always Work

Medicine is an art more than it is a science. Sometimes the recommended treatment doesn't work. It may not work because the dose wasn't correct, or it may not work because the underlying condition causing the symptoms is more severe than originally thought.

Involving Medical Professionals

As is unfortunately usually the case, most physicians will have very little knowledge of CBD*plus*, or medical cannabis. However, it is important to give your doctor the opportunity to assist you controlling your condition. Do not attempt to suddenly decrease or discontinue your prescriptions medications. Involve your doctor, why you gradually titrate the dose of CBD*plus* and other nutraceuticals.

> If your regular doctor won't work with you to dose medical cannabis you can find a compassionate, experienced licensed clinician who will, in your area at the following websites:
>
> www.Leafly.com
>
> www.MarijuanaDoctors.com
>
> www.WeedMaps.com

CHAPTER 10: METABOLIC SYNDROME

Personal Story

> A friend of mine came to see me, as he didn't trust his primary care doctor. He was concerned that his health was "going down the drain." He was only 48 years old, and in the past three years he had been diagnosed with morbid obesity, including a belly "I just can't get rid of, even with loads of exercise."
>
> He then was diagnosed with high blood pressure and high blood fats at his annual physical only a year after that. To make matters worse, he had recently been told he had pre-diabetes and was heading toward diabetes if he didn't "watch out."
>
> After a thorough medical history, including a discussion of his usual diet, his exercise activities and family history of these diseases, I ran a series of tests. Indeed, he had all of the diagnoses that his doctor told him he had. But what he wasn't told was that his underlying problem was metabolic syndrome. He was not falling apart with all sorts of conditions, but had one underlying metabolic issue that was resulting in all of these diagnoses.
>
> We addressed the underlying issue over the next year with dietary changes and nutritional supplements. He changed his exercise routine so that it was more aerobic and supportive of weight loss, and gaining muscle mass. We closely monitored his medications and we were able to take him off of his blood pressure pills and improve his blood sugars and blood fats.

Introduction

Metabolic syndrome is a clustering of at least three of the five medical conditions including abdominal obesity, high blood pressure, high blood sugar, high blood lipids, and/or low high-density lipoprotein (HDL) levels. Some physicians would add non-alcoholic fatty liver disease as a sixth diagnosis, which was discussed in an earlier chapter.

Metabolic syndrome is associated with a substantially increased risk of developing cardiovascular disease and type 2 diabetes. In the United States, nearly a quarter of the adult population has been diagnosed with metabolic syndrome, and has a higher prevalence among increasing age groups as well as racial and ethnic minorities, which are particularly affected.

Insulin resistance, metabolic syndrome, and pre-diabetes are closely related to one another and have many overlapping aspects. Metabolic syndrome is thought to be caused by an underlying disorder of energy (blood sugar) utilization and fat storage but is still an area of ongoing medical research.

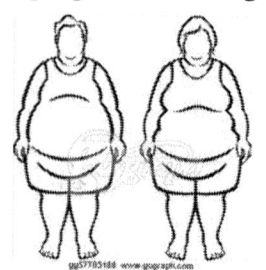

Data provided by the World Health Organization suggests that 65% of the world's population live in countries where overweight lifestyles and obesity kills more people than being underweight does. The W.H.O. defines "overweight" as a BMI greater than or equal to 25, and "obesity" as a BMI greater than or equal to 30. Both overweight and obesity are major risk factors for cardiovascular diseases—specifically heart disease, stroke and diabetes.

The International Diabetes Federation reports that as of 2011, 366 million people suffer from diabetes. This number is projected to increase to over half a billion (estimated 552 million) by 2030.

Several nutraceuticals used in clinical practice have been shown to target the disease processes involved with diabetes mellitus, metabolic syndrome and their complications and to favorably improve the condition and long-term effects. These compounds include antioxidant vitamins such as vitamins C and E, flavonoids, vitamin D, THCV (CBD*plus*), conjugated linoleic acid, omega-3 fatty acids, minerals such as chromium and magnesium, α-lipoic acid, phytoestrogens, and dietary fibers—most of which were discussed in detail in the chapter on weight loss.

Chronic stress and certain "inflammatory" diets have an important role in inflammation that causes type 2 diabetes mellitus and metabolic. With type 2 diabetes, pancreas cell inflammation has been shown to be the underlying mechanism. Oxidative stress from inflammation may also play an important role in the development of complications in diabetes such as lens cataracts, diabetic nephropathy, and diabetic neuropathy.

Animal studies have shown that an adequate supply of dietary antioxidants may prevent or delay diabetes complications including renal and neural dysfunction by providing protection against oxidative stress.

It is important to understand that although insulin and diabetic medications can control several aspects of diabetes, they are oftentimes inadequate for preventing the cardiac and small vessel disease complications that affect the retina, lens, and kidney. Thus, while insulin and diabetic medications—such as metformin—function to improve the elevated blood sugar that comes with diabetes, these drugs might not work to prevent some of the more serious complications also associated with having diabetes. In most cases of diabetes, prescribed medications will be required to maintain adequate blood sugar control; however, the addition of CBD*plus* and several other nutraceuticals—such as anti-oxidant vitamins, fish oils, cinnamon and curcumin--will help fight the effects of metabolic syndrome.

The Conditions that make up Metabolic Syndrome

Obesity and overweight

Diabetes mellitus type 2

Pre-diabetes (insulin resistance)

High blood lipids

High blood pressure

Heart disease

Non-alcoholic fatty liver disease

Increased abdominal girth

Studies of CBD*plus* and Metabolic Syndrome

A study using the National Health and Nutrition Examination Survey (NHANES) was done at the University of Miami in 2015. The researchers found in adults age 20-59 years of age that the "current users" of cannabis had a 54% lower risk of metabolic syndrome than "never" users.

A high-quality clinical study in type 2 diabetes was done in the UK in 2016. The researchers used CBD and THCV (CBD*plus*) together to affect the blood lipid and blood sugar problems seen in the metabolic syndrome. The results showed a decrease in fasting blood sugar, improved pancreatic function, glucose tolerance, adiponectin (which has to do with fat metabolism), and Apo A (the main component of HDL). THCV, both with and without CBD, were noted to be well tolerated among the patients of this clinical study.

Much more research still needs to be done on this hugely important condition. However, based on how safe CBD*plus* is to use, and considering the available evidence is suggestive of a real impact on both the blood sugar and blood lipid metabolic problems that are the foundation of the metabolic syndrome, a preventive dose of 5-20mg twice daily may be appropriate for adults early on in the progression towards full blown metabolic syndrome.

As was discussed in my personal story, CBD*plus* or nutraceuticals do not work in a vacuum. They are part of a well-structured and thought out plan to improve wellness and make life-style changes, that include changes in dietary habits, exercise routines, and often increased mindfulness through yoga or meditation.

Involving Medical Professionals

Unfortunately, it is usually the case that most physicians will have very little knowledge of CBD*plus* and medical cannabis; not to mention, their functions in treating metabolic syndrome, as well. However, it is important to give your doctor the opportunity to assist you in controlling your symptoms. Do not attempt to suddenly decrease or discontinue your prescribed medications. Involve your doctor while you gradually titrate your doses of CBD*plus* and other nutraceuticals.

Sometimes CBD*plus* alone is not enough to get control of the pain and medical cannabis with THC in it will be required. If your regular doctor won't work with you to dose medical cannabis you can find a compassionate, experienced licensed clinician who will, in your area at the following websites:

www.Leafly.com

www.MarijuanaDoctors.com

www.WeedMaps.com

CHAPTER 11: PREVENTIVE DOSES OF CBD*PLUS*

Preventive Doses of CBD*plus*

The available evidence discussed throughout this book shows that CBD*plus*, like CBD, raises the cannabinoid tone in the brain and body. The main net effect of using CBD*plus* on a long-term basis as a preventive medicine would be to maintain healthy blood sugar, blood lipid levels and weight. A secondary benefit would be decreased inflammation in many chronic degenerative diseases that affect us as we age. Table I lists those diseases that have been scientifically associated with chronic inflammation.

Table I
Alzheimer's and other dementias
Cardiovascular diseases, such as heart attack and stroke
Inflammatory-related cancers, such as bowel, prostate, breast and lung
Autoimmune diseases, such as inflammatory arthritis, celiac disease and psoriasis

In addition, long term improved endocannabinoid tone is associated with an improved mood, reduced anxiety and perceived stress.

Ultimately, current societal influences on the ECS results in endocannabinoid deficiency syndromes including irritable bowel syndrome, fibromyalgia, and migraine headache. This deficiency of natural ANA would be improved by the daily use of CBD and CBD*plus*.

This book has also discussed the many studies and clinical observations that confirm the safety of CBD*plus* in adults. Most hemp extracts containing CBD and/or CBD*plus* really could be sold next to olive oil in a grocery store. Therefore, daily use of low doses of CBD and CBD*plus* for preventive purposes are considered completely safe.

Based on the above facts, I recommend a daily dose of 2-5mg a day of CBD*plus* as well as 10-20mg a day of CBD, taken under the tongue once a day.

Always consider adding daily anti-oxidant vitamin, and other anti-oxidant supplements to assistant in preventing the rages of chronic stress and the modern inflammatory diet.

This type of preventive dosing is analogous to the U.S. Preventive Services Task Force recommendation of taking a 81mg dose of aspirin daily to prevent cardiovascular disease and colorectal cancer.

> https://www.uspreventiveservicestaskforce.org/Page/Document/RecommendationStatementFinal/aspirin-to-prevent-cardiovascular-disease-and-cancer

More information -

Go to **www.TheHempDepot.org** and use the COUPON CODE – CANNA-MD171002 for 10% off purchases of whole plant, high quality ABSOLUTE CBD and CBDplus products.

To learn more about the author, his other books, and up-to-date research on CBDplus and medical cannabis go to www.Cannabis-MD.com and www.GregoryLSmithMD.com

ABBREVIATIONS:

11-OH-THC- 11-Hydroxy-THC is the main active metabolite of tetrahydrocannabinol (THC) which is formed in the body after cannabis is consumed. It is more euphoric and potent than THC.

2-AG- 2-Arachidonoylglycerol is one of the body's cannabinoid neurotransmitters. Anandamide (ANA) is the other.

ANA- Anandamide is one of the body's cannabinoid neurotransmitters. 2-AG is the other.

CBD- Cannabidiol, is one of at least 100 cannabinoids identified in cannabis. Like THC and CBG, it is a major phytocannabinoid, accounting for up to 30% of the plant's extract in some strains

CBDV- Cannabidivarin is a very minor cannabinoid. This is the "-varin" version of CBD and is analogous to THCV being the "-varin" version of THC. It works similarly to THCV in many ways.

CBDplus- This is the non-scientific name that the author uses in this book for THCV. Because of the difficult to pronounce name – tetrahydrocannabivarin, and the similarity of THCV to the abbreviation euphoric and addictive THC, the author wanted a name to more aptly represent what this minor cannabinoid does.

CBG- Cannabigerol is one of the minor cannabinoids found in hemp or cannabis oil.

CB1- The cannabinoid receptor type 1 that is primarily found in the brain and on nerve cells.

CB2- The cannabinoid receptor type 2 that is primarily found on immune system cells throughout the body.

CSA- The Controlled Substances Act is the statute establishing federal U.S. drug policy under which the manufacture, importation, possession, use, and distribution of certain substances is regulated. It was established in 1970.

ECS – The endocannabinoid system. This is the system in our brain and body that keeps several other systems in homeostasis or balance. The phrase, "eat, sleep, relax, protect, forget," succinctly summarizes most of the therapeutic effects of the ECS in the brain and body.

FAAH- Fatty acid amide hydrolase is an enzyme. It was first shown to break down anandamide (ANA) in 1993.

FDA- The Food and Drug Administration is a federal agency of the United States Department of Health and Human Services, one of the United States federal executive departments. The FDA is responsible for protecting and promoting public health.

GRAS- Generally recognized as safe is an FDA designation that a chemical or substance added to food is considered safe by experts, and so is exempted from the usual Federal Food, Drug, and Cosmetic Act food additive tolerance requirements.

HDL – High density lipoproteins, generally considered to be the "good" cholesterol.

LDL – Low density lipoproteins, generally considered to be the "bad" cholesterol.

NAFLD – Non-alcoholic fatty liver disease.

PIMSR – Is a C-3 piperidinoiminomethyl is a synthetic analog of Rimonabant, that acts the same as THCV (CBDplus)

RSHO- A brand of hemp oil, that is high in CBD. It is not to be confused with Rick Simpson Oil (RSO), a very potent THC-rich oil for late stage cancer.

RSO- Rick Simpson oil, also known as Phoenix Tears. This is a very potent, THC-rich oil, used in a 90-day regimen for late stage cancer. Requires a physician's supervision.

THC- Tetrahydrocannabinol refers to a psychotropic cannabinoid and is the principal euphoric constituent of cannabis.

Index

"inverse" blocker, 97
"neutral" blocker, 97
"positive" stimulator, 97
11-OH-THC, 30, 63, 167
2014 Farm Bill, 46, 66, 87
2-AG, 53, 54, 56, 97, 131, 134, 167
7-OH-CBD, 63
abdominal obesity, 158
addiction, 1, 28, 42, 44, 51, 82, 87, 96, 100
adipocytes, 136, 139
adiponectin, 116, 137, 161
agitation, 44, 79, 94, 100
alcohol, 10, 40, 45, 63, 76, 77, 82, 92, 93, 96, 151, 152
allergy, 90
ANA, 53, 54, 56, 97, 131, 134, 164, 167, 168
Anandamide, 167
anti-oxidant, 27, 160, 164
anxiety, 44, 73, 82, 89, 94, 100, 129, 132, 163
Apo A, 121, 161
blood lipid, 133, 152, 161, 163
blood sugar, 80, 97, 104, 105, 112, 113, 114, 116, 117, 131, 132, 133, 136, 137, 140, 142, 147, 152, 158, 160, 161, 163
blood-brain barrier, 136
BMI, 125, 126, 127, 158
Body Mass Index, 125
breast milk, 92
cannabidivarin, 4, 9, 59, 138
cannabinoid tone, 163
Cannabis butter, 78
CannaKit, 71
carbon dioxide (CO2) extraction., 33
catechin, 144
CB1, 53, 54, 56, 57, 58, 59, 60, 66, 82, 97, 101, 120, 128, 129, 131, 132, 133, 134, 135, 137, 138, 153, 154, 155, 167
CB2, 25, 53, 54, 56, 58, 59, 60, 66, 97, 101, 153, 154, 155, 168
CBC, 9, 29, 83
CBDV, 4, 9, 15, 43, 59, 60, 92, 138, 167
CBG,, 83, 167
CBN, 9, 30, 83
Children, 93
chlorogenic acid, 148
cholesterol, 119, 120, 121, 122, 126, 131, 132, 133, 142, 168
chromium, 146, 147, 159
chromodulin, 146
chronic stress, 164

cinnamaldehyde, 140, 141
cinnamon, 139, 140, 141, 142, 143, 160
coffee, 148
COMT, 143
Consistency, 88
Contaminants, 88
curcumin, 139, 140, 147, 160
dependency, 8, 51, 87, 96
depression, 97, 132, 133
diabetic medications, 160
dietary supplement, 149
dopamine, 135
drug test, 107
ECS, 7, 15, 24, 27, 29, 43, 48, 51, 52, 53, 55, 57, 59, 60, 61, 84, 85, 93, 95, 108, 128, 131, 136, 138, 164, 168
elderly, 94
entourage effect', 27
Epidiolex, 14, 47, 48, 83, 84
euphoria, 1, 7, 8, 9, 10, 24, 25, 28, 31, 51, 60, 72, 81, 82, 87, 89, 90, 94, 95, 100
extraction techniques, 32, 76, 87
FAAH-, 168
fat metabolism, 151, 161
FDA, 14, 47, 48, 87, 91, 94, 97, 106, 128, 168
fiber supplements, 149

fibromyalgia, 164
flavonoids, 27, 76, 159
Gestational diabetes, 113
ghrelin, 135, 136
glucomannan, 148
Green tea, 143
GTE, 143
gut flora, 144, 145
hair growth, 82
HDL, 120, 121, 131, 132, 133, 158, 161, 168
hepatic fibrosis, 154
high blood pressure, 126, 157, 158
hyperlipidemia, 119, 120, 139
hypothalamus, 135, 136
inflammation, 58, 59, 60, 62, 65, 84, 151, 159, 163
infused topicals, 82
insulin, 112, 113, 115, 116, 131, 132, 133, 139, 142, 146, 151, 160
irritable bowel syndrome, 59, 164
LDL, 119, 121, 131, 133, 142, 168
leptin, 131, 136
liver disease, 153, 154
liver enzymes, 152
MDI, 71
metabolic syndrome, 132, 142, 149, 151, 157, 158, 159, 160, 161, 162

methylhydroxychalcone polymer, 142
micro-dose inhaler, 71
migraine, 164
mood, 89, 94, 95, 104, 129, 163
munchies, 1, 57, 134
NAFLD, 151, 168
nausea, 42, 60, 97, 129, 131, 134
NIDDM, 113
non-alcoholic fatty liver disease, 151, 158
Non-alcoholic fatty liver disease, 160, 168
nucleus accumbens, 135
Oromuscosal absorption, 78
oxidative stress, 61, 159
P450, 94, 95
pancreatic, 116, 139, 141, 161
panic, 79
paranoia, 44, 96
PIMSR, 133, 152, 169
pre-biotic, 146
Pre-diabetes, 2, 113, 160
pregnancy, 91, 92
ProCon.org, 16, 108
psychosis, 96
psyllium, 148

Rick Simpson oil, 169
Rimonabant, 97, 115, 128, 129, 130, 131, 132, 138, 169
schizophrenia, 96
short-term memory, 94, 100
silymarin, 155
spices, 139
Start Low, Go Slow, 100
stomach rumbling, 135, 136, 138
suicidal thoughts, 97, 132
suicide, 97, 128, 129
terpenes, 23, 24, 25, 27, 31, 32, 62, 68, 74, 76, 83, 84, 103
Tetrahydrocannabinol, 28, *169*
topical preparations, 82
turmeric, 139
type 2 diabetes, 121, 126, 146, 158, 159, 161
weight loss, 97, 102, 104, 112, 115, 128, 131, 133, 138, 143, 145, 148, 151, 152, 157, 159
whole plant extract, 70, 83, 84

Made in the USA
Columbia, SC
13 October 2018